TO BE A NURSE

LINDA STRANGIO, RN, MA, CCRN

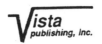
Vista publishing, Inc.

Edited by Lisa Ruggerio, RN and Carolyn S. Zagury, MS, RN, CPC

Cover design by Thomas Taylor of Thomcatt Graphics

Vista Publishing, Inc.
473 Broadway
Long Branch, NJ 07740
(908) 229-6500

This publication is written for the reading pleasure of the general public. The author is solely responsible for the content of the written work and has fictionalized the stories, characters, and places in this publication in order to protect any issues of confidentiality.

Printed and bound in the United States of America

First Edition

ISBN: 1-880254-22-0

Library of Congress Catalog Card Number: 94-61761

U.S.A. Price $12.95
Canada Price $17.95

DEDICATION

. . . . . To my Concentrated Care and Surgical I.C.U. families, who
taught me what it means to be a real nurse.

. . . . . To my new Radiology family, who made me once again look
forward to coming to work every day.

. . . . . To all my patients and their families, who have allowed me the
privilege of becoming a small part of their lives.

. . . . . To my mother, who would have been so proud.

Thank you.

SPECIAL THANKS

I want to thank Dr. Harriet Forman, Executive Director of *Nursing Spectrum*, for her help and encouragement. I saved a letter in which she wrote to me, "Continue to write. You have touching and interesting things to say, and you say them with heart." These words helped me when I didn't know if I should keep on trying to put this book together.

Thank you to the staff of *Nursing Spectrum* for printing some of my stories and then for releasing them so I could include them in this book.

Thanks to my husband, Vinny, who finally convinced me to switch from my typewriter to the computer and then taught me how to use it.

I also want to thank Carol Larkin, my best friend, who let me read every single story to her over the phone and critiqued them all. (Actually, she wasn't very much of a critic, since she said every one was absolutely wonderful!).

And I especially thank Carolyn Zagury, who believed in me enough to make my dream of becoming a writer when I grew up come true.

MEET THE AUTHOR

Linda Strangio was born in Brooklyn, and graduated from The Mount Sinai Hospital School of Nursing in New York City. She received a bachelors degree in psychology from Caldwell College and a masters degree in industrial and organizational psychology from Montclair State University, both in New Jersey.

Linda holds national certification in critical care nursing (C.C.R.N.) and spent many years as a staff nurse, head nurse, and patient care coordinator in the intensive care units. For the past few years, she has been the nursing coordinator for the Department of Radiology at The Mountainside Hospital in Montclair, New Jersey. She is a frequent contributor to nursing journals and magazines, and is a member of several professional organizations.

The mother of three grown children, Linda lives with her husband in Glen Ridge, New Jersey. She enjoys knitting, crocheting, bowling, and doing crossword puzzles. Linda especially loves throwing quarters into the Atlantic city slot machines, where she knows that one day soon, she is going to hit "the big one."

TABLE OF CONTENTS

TABLE OF CONTENTS

TABLE OF CONTENTS

INTRODUCTION

This book is a collection of true stories, stories of years and years of experiences in hospitals. The patients and incidents are real or are composites of real people and events. Although the names have been changed, the facts and emotions have not.

The stories in this book are based on compilations of many different people, places and events. Some happened just as they are portrayed, while others are put together from multiple events, experiences, and varied health care settings. Names of the characters are fictitious and the incidents described are not representative of any particular hospital.

These are stories that show just what it means *To Be A Nurse*. Some are funny and some are sad. Some end happy and others don't. But, all of them are about *the special people who have chosen the finest of all helping professions.*

PROLOGUE

It seems as if I've always been a nurse. The hospital bug has been in my blood for so long that it's a part of what I am. A very big part. I've never really been away from nursing, except for a few months during my three maternity leaves. And each time that I came back, I realized how much I had missed it. Even for those couple of months. And now thirty years later, I still love being a nurse. A hospital nurse.

Over the years there have been so many changes in the way nursing is practiced. When I try to remember how we did things back then, it seems hard to believe that was truly the state of the art. The starched bibs and aprons I wore as a student nurse and the big old open wards I worked on seem like parts of scenes from old movies. But that was my life, and I loved it then the same as I do now.

When I became a nurse, it was during a time when most women who wanted careers either turned to teaching or nursing. Lots of kids in my high school senior class went on to nursing school. It was the thing to do. For girls, anyway. There were no male nurses. At least I never knew any.

Many years ago, when I first became a nurse we mixed antibiotics, vitamins, and everything else together in glass I.V. bottles. There were no piggy backs or thoughts of drug compatibility. We started our I.V.'s with number 18 metal needles. There were no angiocaths. At the end of the shift, we spent time in the utility room where we washed, wrapped and labeled nasogastric tubes, foleys, red rubber catheters, and glass syringes to be autoclaved. There were no disposables. Everything was reused for the next patient.

Penicillin was "the drug" and we used huge doses. Twenty million units in each I.V. bottle three times a day was routine. We made beds with rubber sheets; there were no chux. There was no paper tape or silk tape--just plain old white adhesive, and if the patient's skin got red, we moved the tape. There were no trays or kits for anything; we made our own. We used silver emesis basins and round bowls to hold all our equipment. When we gave injections, we combined several drugs in one syringe. If the medication didn't turn white and get hard, we gave the shot. When the patients were discharged, we carbolized their beds. We were the housekeepers also. That was part of nursing.

There were no care plans. We just followed the doctors' orders without question. In fact, I remember having to stand up and give up our chairs to the doctors when they came into the nurses' station. And they took them!

Foleys drained into plastic bags attached to wire racks. If we ran out of bags, we stuck the ends of the drainage tubes into empty glass I.V. bottles. Nobody knew about closed systems or infection control practices. I can remember making rounds on a large G.U. ward, irrigating all thirty foley catheters and never washing my hands until I was all finished. And maybe not even then.

The routine equipment we take for granted today wasn't even a dream when I first began to practice nursing. I.V. infusion pumps and electronic thermometers, heparin locks and multi-lumen catheters, hypothermia blankets and even electric call bells were all things of the future. All I.V. fluids ran through the same I.V. tubing which stayed up for the duration of the hospital stay.

I became an I.C.U. nurse back when the concept of intensive care first began. In those days, that meant we put the sickest patients together and did the most to them. We learned to read cardiac monitors as we worked, since there were no critical care courses or certifications. We could see the monitors, but had no print-outs. There were no paste-on leads, so we attached them with number 25 gauge needles subcutaneously and held the needles in place with tape. (They didn't seem to hurt!)

We worked exclusively with Bird respirators; there were no volume cycled respirators then. We made ventilator changes by looking at and listening to the patients, since there were no arterial blood gases. There were no CT scanners or MRI's, so craniotomies were rarely done for intracerebral bleeds. Carotid endarterectomies and open heart surgery had very high mortality rates. All patients with poor veins had cut-downs, and many of these became quickly infected.

There were no invasive monitoring techniques. What was a Swan-Ganz or a temporary pacemaker wire? Patients with flail chests had their broken ribs grasped with towel clips and hooked to traction for about a week or so. All major upper G.I. bleeds were treated by passing gastric hypothermia balloons through the mouth which stayed in place and circulated chilled alcohol through the big hoses. And they stayed in for days. We lost almost every single CPR patient, since the technique was so new and there was no such thing as code protocol. Many doctors believed that if closed chest CPR failed, they were obligated to open the chest. We did quite a few bedside thoracotomies. Just a little messy.

When patients were admitted, they signed consent for whatever needed to be done. There were no consents for special procedures, and all operative permits allowed "any surgery deemed necessary." Families were considered to be a burden to patient care. Patients' rights and ethical dilemmas were not addressed, since the hospital and its staff always knew best. Nurses had no continuing education, no quality assurance, and of course no certifications.

But we still cared about and cared for our patients. Maybe on paper it didn't show like it does now, but we still wanted to make things better. We didn't want people to be hurt or to be sick or to be afraid. That part of nursing has never changed and it never will. We've come a long way in nursing, and in years to come, the way we practice will continue to be dramatically different. But the basics and the caring will never change. And that, truly, is what it means to be a nurse.

TO BE A REAL NURSE

He was ringing that bell again. Every 10 minutes she'd hear, "I'm hot. I'm cold. Raise my head. Lower me. Give me a drink." Karen had two other patients in the intensive care unit to care for besides Mr. Garibaldi. Both were on ventilators, and both were really sick.

Mr. Garibaldi was relatively stable now. He had suffered serious facial injuries in an auto accident and had been in and out of congestive heart failure during the time he was on a ventilator. But now he was almost ready to be transferred out of the unit. He was receiving small amounts of humidified oxygen through his tracheostomy and was awake and alert. Karen knew he didn't want to leave the security of the ICU.

There went the bell again. Karen was changing intravenous tubing in the next room. Mr. Garibaldi would just have to wait for a few minutes, she thought. Everyone else is busy, and I can't keep running in there every 10 minutes. As she left Mrs. Browning's bedside a few minutes later, she could hear the gurgling. It sounded like bubbles of air moving through water. And that's exactly what it was. Mr. Garibaldi was in raging pulmonary edema.

It's all my fault, thought Karen. He felt it coming on. He knew something was wrong. That's why he was ringing the bell so often. I should have known better. As she suctioned Mr. Garibaldi and gave him Lasix, she tried to talk to him and calm him down. "It's OK. It's OK," she repeated. But who was she really talking to, him or herself? And was it really OK? Karen felt terrible and ashamed.

The next day when she arrived at work, Mr. Garibaldi looked great. He was in normal sinus rhythm and his color was pink. Karen felt better and even more so when Mr. Garibaldi gave her a big wave and a smile.

About 10:30AM, Mr. Garibaldi put his light on. Karen went right in, and as soon as she saw him, she knew what happened. Mr. Garibaldi was sitting on the side of his bed looking absolutely panic stricken. His color was dusky and his skin was cool and moist. His heart rate was rapid and he was gesturing wildly to his throat. He could no longer speak by placing his finger over the tracheostomy opening. In fact, Karen noted that almost no air was moving through that airway.

Karen knew that dried mucus or a blood plug had occluded Mr. Garibaldi's airway. She knew that his facial edema still prevented an effective oral or nasal air exchange. She also knew that this was a true emergency because unless she could clear his airway, Mr. Garibaldi could suffocate.

After calling for help, Karen quickly grabbed the suction catheter and attempted to insert it into the tracheostomy tube. The catheter would not pass. The cuff was already flat, so Karen pulled out the inner cannula in the hope that the blockage was there. It wasn't. She again tried to push the suction catheter down and once again she was unable to do so.

By that time, another nurse and a respiratory therapist were at the bedside trying to help. Karen grabbed a prepackaged dose of sterile normal saline. She broke off the tip and squirted the fluid into the tracheostomy tube to try to dissolve the occlusion. Again Karen tried to pass the suction catheter. No good.

Mr. Garibaldi was becoming combative and disoriented. His skin color was getting worse as he fought for air. Now he needed to be physically restrained so that the staff could work on him. Two nurses restrained him as Karen grabbed the ambu bag and tried to force air into his lungs.

Finally, Karen felt something give way. Mr. Garibaldi began to cough and Karen removed the bag. A hard reddish brown plug shot out of the tracheostomy tube. Mr. Garibaldi began to breathe and his color came back. He was OK.

After suctioning Mr. Garibaldi a few more times to make sure there were no more plugs , Karen placed him back on humidified oxygen. With his face still distorted and swollen from the incident, he smiled a crooked smile and put both his soaking wet arms around Karen and hugged her.

"Thank you," he whispered, as he covered the opening of the tracheostomy tube. "I'll never forget what you did for me. You are a very special nurse." No, Mr. Garibaldi, Karen said to herself. Thank you. Karen felt good again.

"To Be A Real Nurse," by Linda Strangio, RN, MA, CCRN as reprinted with permission of The *Nursing Spectrum*, New York/New Jersey Metro Edition, Vol. 3, No. 6, July, 1993.

SECTION ONE

MIRACLES

SHE WAS ONLY NINETEEN

She was a tall, beautiful young lady, but her skin had taken on that waxy tinge so indicative of an impending ominous medical event. Her hands and feet were blue. The constant temperatures of 104 to 105 degrees kept her body core hot and her extremities cold. Her mouth, no matter how often the nurses cleaned it, was dry and crusty. Her eyes were half open, and her head was bent to the side. She was deep in coma.

Helena had been admitted just a few days before with a virulent form of encephalitis. She was responsive on admission, but the outlook appeared grim when she lost consciousness that first night. She no longer responded to stimulation - not even deep pain.

Helena's family situation was a tragedy in itself. Her parents had come to America from a third world country when she was a child. Her father had been left behind in a prison camp, and her older brother had been killed in a bus accident. All that was left of this family was Helena and her mother.

Helena's prognosis was listed as grave, with virtually no hope offered. The physicians believed that if Helena were to recover, she would surely have begun to show improvement by now. The staff expected her to arrest at any time.

About 9 pm on a Saturday evening, Helena's mother was in the big soft chair in the corner, staring out the window. Cathy, who had been Helena's nurse for the past three nights, was at the bedside changing one of the many intravenous tubings. The room was lit only by the light of the monitors, pumps, and screens.

"Ma, I have a headache," Helena suddenly whined. Her mother jumped to her feet screaming in amazement. Cathy let out a whoop, grabbing Helena's mother in a bear hug. They both burst into tears.

Everything went nuts. Staff members ran in: everyone was laughing, crying, and clapping. Helena's mother ran out of the medical intensive care unit, into the surgical ICU, and then through the telemetry area. She threw her arms around everyone she met, hugging them and screaming in elation. People started to follow her, and by the time she returned to Helena's bedside, it looked like a parade.

Helena was sweating like crazy; her fever began to break. She was holding her head, sitting up, and looking totally bewildered. Was this a miracle? We think so.

"She Was Only Nineteen," by Linda Strangio, RN, MA, CCRN, as reprinted with permission of *The Nursing Spectrum*, New York/New Jersey Metro Edition, Vol. 5, No. 2, January 25, 1993.

THE MIRACLE BABY

They has been married for almost twenty years and had no children. The fact was that Mrs. Nelson had been labeled infertile after many years of trying to become pregnant. Resigned to the fact that they would always be a family of two, the Nelsons lived their lives fully and happily. They both had good jobs, loved to travel, and had lots of nieces and nephews to love. Life was, after all, pretty good.

The month after her fortieth birthday, Mrs. Nelson found a lump in her breast. It looked benign, her doctor said, but just to be on the safe side it was better to remove it. The bomb fell on all of them when the pathology report came back. It was malignant. So the next step was to have some more surgery and remove the lymph glands under Mrs. Nelson's arm, and that was done soon after. This time the bomb was even bigger. She had three nodes which had been infiltrated with cancer cells.

So Mrs. Nelson began her chemotherapy treatments to try to kill any remaining cancer and save her life. And she didn't have a very easy time of it either. If there ever was a side effect from the chemo, Mrs. Nelson had it. You name it. Vomiting, sores in her mouth, fevers from the low blood counts, etc. If the books said it could happen, it happened to Mrs. Nelson. And of course she lost her beautiful hair. Unable to work because of all her side effects, Mrs. Nelson took a medical leave of absence. Her future was, at best, uncertain.

Then, Mrs. Nelson noticed that her abdomen was beginning to become bloated. It seemed that over a period of just a few months, her belly had become big and swollen. She felt, she said, the fluid shifting around in there, and it was getting harder to breathe. Her oncologist sat down with her and her husband and had a heart to heart talk with them. It looked very much as if the cancer had spread to the liver and elsewhere in the abdomen, he told them, and that was a very poor sign. Obviously this meant that all the months of that terrible chemotherapy hadn't worked after all. Mrs. Nelson needed to have an abdominal CT scan to find the extent of the cancer.

On the morning of the scan, Mrs. Nelson arrived in the radiology department holding back tears. She knew she would know, in a very short time, whether or not she was going to die. She was scared to death, and so was her husband. Mrs. Nelson came into the scanning room and lay down while the technologist took what they call a scout or a preliminary film.

The control room was busy and nobody was paying much attention until suddenly the technologist called out loud to show people what she was seeing on her monitor screen. There, among all the abdominal organs in Mrs. Nelson's abdomen, was a fetus. A big fetus, about seven months old. That was what had made Mrs. Nelson's belly get so big, and that was what was moving around. It wasn't a tumor or abdominal fluid, but a baby.

Everyone gathered around the one monitor to see the baby, this baby who had grown inside a lady who had been fed poisons for the past several months. "Oh, my God," everyone kept saying over and over again. "Oh, my God." Someone ran to get a radiologist who came in to see this miracle which had grown out of that deadly environment. "How are we going to tell her?" someone asked. "Who knows what this baby is like?"

The radiologist and one of the nurses opened the door and went into the scanning room. "Mrs. Nelson," the radiologist said seriously. "We know why your abdomen has gotten so big." Mrs. Nelson braced herself, waiting to hear the death sentence of a big metastatic tumor. "You have a baby in there. A big baby." Mrs. Nelson looked at the doctor, not seeming to understand what he was saying to her. He repeated the CT scan findings two more times. "How did this happen?" asked Mrs. nelson, almost in shock. "Oh, the usual way, I guess," laughed the radiololgist. Mrs. Nelson did not laugh.

"What about the baby?" she asked. "How could the baby be all right with all those medicines I took?" The radiologist just shook his head. "Let's go over to the ultrasound department and see just what this baby looks like," he said softly. "Do you want me to tell your husband?" Mrs. Nelson just shook her head. "Let me tell him," she said sadly.

Mrs. Nelson, still in her examination gown, climbed off the table and walked out of the room right into the waiting area. She silently took her husband by the hand and led him into an empty office and closed the door. About ten minutes later, they emerged, both in tears. The husband was shaking all over.

The staff took Mrs. Nelson down to the the ultrasound department, and a sonogram was done right then and there. Two radiologists stood by to the tell the family the bad news, but they and everyone else were absolutely shocked. This baby, which had been fed poisons and chemicals all of its life, seemed perfectly normal and healthy. If appeared fully formed and was moving around just like any seven month old fetus.

So the Nelsons went home and the oncologist, who was notified by phone of his unknown patient, almost had a heart attack right then and there. After some quick figuring it turned out that the chemotherapy had begun at around the eighth week of gestation, just missing the time when the baby's vital organs were forming. So that baby, although getting some anesthesia during Mrs. Nelson's surgery, just missed the time when the poisons given to his mom could do the most damage to him.

Well, Mrs. Nelson's chemotherapy was stopped immediately and, without its side effects, she soon began to feel great. Her hair grew back and she developed a voracious appetite and started to gain weight. She spent the last two months of her pregnancy being treated by a group of doctors who specialize in high risk deliveries. And a big eight pound healthy miracle baby boy was born to Mrs. Nelson, during an easy normal delivery.

That was almost two years ago. Mrs. Nelson's cancer remains in full remission, and the fat little baby is now a healthy toddler right in the middle of his "terrible twos". Time will tell whether or not some problem will surface years down the road, but for now this family is counting its blessings. Somebody up there is watching over them.

MIRACLES ARE MADE OF THIS

Viola Morgan had been involved in a minor car accident - a simple "fender bender." Although it was the type of accident that usually causes nothing more than a whiplash, Mrs. Morgan had broken her neck. Her spinal cord was irreparably damaged at the level of C2 - an injury that could lead to sudden death. When patients survive, they may not be able to breathe, speak, or swallow. And, certainly, all voluntary movement below the neck is lost.

Mrs. Morgan surprised us all by not succumbing to this terrible injury. We hadn't anticipated a positive outcome; after all, she was 72 years old. We placed her on a rotor-rest bed with 10 pounds of weight attached to the tongs drilled into the sides of her head. In addition to the multiple monitors and indwelling lines and catheters, she had a tracheostomy. Mrs. Morgan was unable to breathe at all on her own, so the ventilator delivered a predetermined 12 breaths per minute.

To our amazement, Mrs. Morgan remained awake, alert, and oriented. She felt no pain. The damage to her spinal cord had also ended all sensory function.

So here it was, early Easter morning. A devout Catholic, Mrs. Morgan was watching Easter Mass on television. Lauren approached her bedside to hang a new intravenous bag and stopped short. The orange "assist" light was flashing on the ventilator; Mrs. Morgan was breathing.

Lauren looked at Mrs. Morgan's chest and counted the breaths - 40 per minute. They were shallow, but they were breaths, and they were enough to signal the assist light.

This is physically impossible, Lauren told herself. Mrs. Morgan cannot breathe alone. She went out to get another nurse. "Am I cracking up," asked Lauren, "or is she breathing?" She was breathing all right. The respiratory therapist and the residents came to see. They took her off the ventilator for a full minute and she kept right on breathing. They put her back on, and that orange assist light began to flash again. Mrs. Morgan just smiled.

When the Mass was over, Mrs. Morgan stopped breathing on her own. The orange assist light never went on again, and nobody ever saw her take another breath. The ventilator continued to give her 12 breaths per minute until she was transferred to a nursing home, where she would remain for the rest of her life. What happened during that Easter Sunday early morning hour? Nobody really knows.

"Miracles Are Made of This," by Linda Strangio, RN, MA, CCRN is reprinted with permission of *The Nursing Spectrum*, New York/New Jersey Metro Edition, Vol. 5A, No. 21, p. NJ-6, July 26, 1993.

THE SURPRISE

She was seven and a half months pregnant and she had appendicitis. They had to operate before the appendix burst. There was no time to waste. So she went into the operating room and her husband and parents waited anxiously to see if she and the baby would be all right.

As hoped, the surgery went fine and the doctor came out to tell the family the good news. Helen would be in the recovery room for a few hours and then she would go to her room. Go have a cup of coffee and relax, they were told. Come upstairs in about two hours and you can see her before you go home.

Now this happened a few years ago, when things were a little bit different. First of all, the recovery room closed at ten o'clock and no nurses were on call. So, the step-down unit functioned as the makeshift recovery room, and patients who needed surgery at night were placed in the middle of the unit to react. There was an area with oxygen and suction, and these patients were placed on the portable cardiac monitor only if they were unstable.

Also, fetal monitors were not used for pregnant patients. The routine was to listen to the fetal heart once a shift and if the nurses had problems or questions, they called the obstetrical nurses for answers. That's the way things were done and there never had been any problems.

So Helen was rolled out from the operating room right into the step-down unit. She was partially reacted from anesthesia and the anesthesiologist gave the nurses report. It was after midnight. The patient was fine and so was the baby, he said. The surgery was just in time, since the appendix was on the verge of rupturing. But, no problems were expected and it had turned out to be a routine case.

Yeah, right.

Almost as soon as the doctor left the unit, Helen started to moan and complain of abdominal pain. She was now wide awake and becoming very restless. This must really hurt, thought JoAnn, who was taking care of her. She imagined the weight of the baby and the pregnant uterus pushing against the fresh surgical site. Ouch.

JoAnn checked the orders and sure enough, there was one for some Demerol. She really needs this, said JoAnn to herself, as she gave Helen her injection. After about five minutes Helen calmed sown. Good, thought JoAnn. It worked.

But ten minutes later Helen started moaning again, and this time she seemed to be in worse pain. Helen became very restless and was crying out loud.

Hey, what's going on here, wondered JoAnn. At that minute Helen kicked off her sheet and there right between her legs was the top of a baby's head.

Now the last delivery JoAnn had seen was twenty years ago, when she was in nursing school, and at that time she was just an innocent observer. Tonight it was a bit different.

At first JoAnn froze. She just stood there thinking that this couldn't be happening. How could a woman have a baby in a hospital filled with doctors and nurses and end up being left alone with a nurse who didn't know a placenta from an umbilical cord?

"Betty!" screamed JoAnn. "Come help me!" She ran over to the linen cart and grabbed a bath towel. Remember, back then gloves were not kept by every bedside as they are now. This was long before the days of universal precautions. So, as Betty came running out of the medication room, JoAnn's big contribution to this delivery was to lay the bath towel in the bed, over the bloody sheets between Helen's legs. By this time, Betty was on the phone to the delivery room.

Within a minute, that little seven month baby was out of Helen, and lying on the trusty bath towel. The baby was crying and moving his arms and legs, which even JoAnn knew to be a good sign. She just stood there, afraid to try to pick up the baby since the long umbilical cord attached to him was still inside his mother. As long as the kid was breathing, everything was O.K., JoAnn reasoned to herself. Besides, she was shaking so hard that she knew if she even touched that baby she probably would give him a fractured skull or something.

At that time, two delivery room nurses came in right through the swinging doors. One had some kind of a kit with her and another was pushing an Isolette. They were all business and totally calm. As JoAnn later put it, one nurse opened that kit and went "clamp, clamp, snip" and the cord was cut. That nurse just picked up the baby in some kind of sheet or towel and wiped his face and mouth. The other nurse took care of Helen and before anyone knew it, the placenta came right out.

Two other nurses came in at that minute. JoAnn guessed they were from the nursery or the post-partum floor or some place else in maternity. With a big smile, they took Helen away, promising they would bring her back in a little while.

JoAnn sat down in a chair at the nurses' station. Everything had happened so fast, she almost thought she was dreaming. Betty and another nurse called the supervisor and the doctors and took care of the details. It took JoAnn a while to get herself together.

They kept Helen in the O.B. recovery room for a few hours, and the baby boy was sent out to a newborn intensive care unit. Besides his small size, he looked fine and none the worse for coming into this world with JoAnn as his midwife.

It was decided to keep Helen as a patient in that same step-down unit. After all, she was still a post-op patient. When Helen returned a few hours later, the private room was ready. There was a big sign outside the door reading,

"IT'S A BOY!"

Naturally, the sign was made by Betty, since JoAnn had done enough in the way of creativity that night.

When the day staff arrived the next morning there was another sign outside the unit.

"WE HAD A BABY!"

the sign announced. JoAnn and the entire unit were celebrities for quite some time.

MOTHER'S DAY

When she arrived at work that Monday after Mother's Day, the cake was there. She knew it would be. A big chocolate covered sheet cake with pink gooey flowers, it had the usual *THANK YOU* printed in icing right in the middle. Gina smiled to herself as one of the newer nurses asked where the cake had come from.

She'd never forget that Mother's Day fourteen years ago. She was filling in as the weekend supervisor that morning and had gotten report about the kid who was dying up in the I.C.U. He was only twenty-one years old and had been involved in a terrible auto accident the night before. With multiple internal injuries, a flail chest, and many fractures, it was the massive head injury that was probably going to kill him.

Peter was a big handsome boy, over six feet and weighing two hundred thirty pounds. He was a weight lifter and Gina remembered that at first she thought both of his IV's had badly infiltrated into his arms until she realized those bulges were his big muscles. That stuck out in her memory as her first impression of Peter.

Peter's mother was by his bedside, just staring at him. She wasn't crying; in fact, she had no expression on her face. She was numb. Peter was totally unresponsive, on a ventilator, and with tubes going in and coming out of everywhere. Even though he had been cleaned up, his many abrasions oozed slowly onto the clean linen. Peter's eyes were swollen shut.

Two by two, Gina brought the family in to say good-bye. There must have been twenty-five people. Besides his mom and dad and two sisters, there were aunts and uncles and cousins and two grandmothers. Each one touched him and kissed him and told him they loved him. She could feel the love in the room, as much as she felt the deep sadness and the sense of loss. There was no talk of brain death or organ donation back then. It was just a time to say good-bye.

Gina was very conscious of the Mother's Day corsage she wore. If she had thought of it, she would have taken it off before she had come up to the unit, but it was too late. She thought it would look worse if she removed it now. Someone would probably notice. But she felt so guilty, as if she had something to celebrate on this Mother's Day and they didn't.

Well, that day passed and so did the next. Then suddenly it was the Sunday after Mother's Day and Peter was still there. Ever so slowly, Peter started to respond. It wasn't like the movies where patients are in deep comas and suddenly they open their eyes and are wide awake. But Peter got better. His surgical tubes came out and he was weaned off the respirator. And, most of all, Peter became Peter again.

Three months later and seventy pounds lighter, Peter left the hospital. Being a weight lifter, he was used to exercise and looked forward to all his rehabilitation. He knew he'd make a full recovery.

Gina got a long letter that week from Peter's mother, addressed to her care of the nursing office. Peter's mother told her that through that horrible first day, she was aware of Gina and how kind she was to all the family members, giving all of them the time they needed to say good-bye to their very special boy. She also said she remembered the corsage and how somehow seeing Gina wear it made her feel that Gina understood what only another mother could.

Nine months later, on the next Mother's Day, Peter and his mother came up to the I.C.U. where Peter had spent those first weeks. They had a big sheet cake for the nursing staff with words - *THANK YOU*. Peter had gained back almost all of his weight and he looked, once again, like a big strong body builder. He remembered nothing of the unit or the staff, but he thanked everyone for taking care of him. His mom never stopped smiling.

To this day, Peter's mother comes to the intensive care unit every Mother's Day with that big chocolate cake. She doesn't know any of the nurses there today, but that doesn't make any difference to her. It is her way of saying thank you for the miracle.

LIFE AND DEATH

The call for the pediatric code had triggered the usual feeling of dread throughout the hospital. It is never the same as a routine cardiac arrest call which brings the rush of adrenalin in the code teams. No, this was always different. A pediatric code gives everyone a sick feeling. Kids are never supposed to die.

This time, the patient wasn't yet in the house, but was on her way in, with CPR in progress. It was most likely a S.I.D.S. baby. The paramedics had alerted the emergency department by radio, and now the whole hospital was ready. All the floors had heard the call and so did the departments. Housekeepers, dietary workers, and maintenance men all waited for the word. The news always spreads quickly in a hospital.

Although the emergency department usually handles its own codes, it's different with a child. Respiratory therapists, E.K.G. people, nursery and pediatric nurses, and the in-house pediatricians and neonatologists came too. Everyone waited.

The mobile I.C.U. arrived a few minutes later and the baby was wheeled in with the CPR still going on. They were doing mouth to mouth and two finger chest compressions. The little girl was two weeks old. The parents followed behind, assisted by the emergency room personnel. They were in shock.

So the code continued, led by one of the pediatricians. It lasted a very long time. The parents were allowed to see their baby at various intervals during the frantic effort to save her. Several times the mother cried out that if her baby didn't make it, she wanted to make sure that her organs were given to another child.

The baby's heartbeat finally came back but she never began to breathe on her own. Her pupils were fixed and dilated. A pediatric I.C.U. transport team was on the way to take the baby, who was on a little Cub respirator, to a large children's center. The prognosis was terrible. The parents, heartbroken, were with their baby. When the team came they left together for the children's hospital.

As the family and transport team left, the feeling of sadness and despair in the emergency department was almost unbearable. Everyone felt an overwhelming sense of loss. It was a tragedy.

Just then the main doors to the emergency department swung open and a young woman in a wheelchair rolled in, being pushed by a wide-eyed young man. "My wife is having a baby!" he yelled. She sure was. In fact, the baby was partially out already, right between her legs in that wheelchair.

The staff grabbed the handles of the chair and ran right into the O.B. room. Three people lifted the patient up onto the table and thirty seconds later, a new little baby was screaming and crying at the top of her lungs. And, of course, it was a girl.

The tears of sadness in that E.R. turned to those of joy. That staff had gone from sending an almost dead baby girl away, to immediately bringing a newborn baby girl into this world. And it felt like a miracle had occurred.

The next day, the first hospital learned that the little S.I.D.S. baby had died, but her organs had been harvested to save another baby's life. Her heart was transplanted into a baby with not more than a day left to live. And the new heart started to beat immediately and perfectly.

So life had won out after all. One baby had died but two had lived. Somehow that made things easier.

JUST LOOK AT HIM NOW

Judy was Bob's primary nurse for the full six weeks that he was a patient in the surgical I.C.U. She, along with the rest of the staff, never believed that Bob would live. But if he did live, they all felt he would remain hopelessly brain damaged.

After all, Bob's aortic aneurysm had ruptured while he was on the CAT scan table just an hour after he had come into the emergency department complaining of severe abdominal and back pains. According to the radiology staff, they had actually watched this thing blow right there on the computer screens and had rushed him right from the CT department to the operating room. Twenty-two units of blood later, Bob was brought to the S.I.C.U. in extremely guarded condition.

Just about everything that could happen to a patient like this did happen. The loss of blood to the kidneys ended all renal function. His clotting factors were affected and he bled continuously. He needed ventilator assistance to breathe. He developed repeated bouts of pulmonary edema. He became septic. He had intractable, dehydrating diarrheas. And so on.

It was hard to truly evaluate Bob's level of consciousness, since he needed various intravenous paralytic agents to keep him from fighting the respirator. Even with meticulous eye care, his right eye swelled and dried out, so much so, that Judy knew that they could not even use his corneas for donation when the time came that Bob finally died. It was not a question of "if" he died, but rather "when" he died.

Bob was only fifty years old and his wife, Marcy, was his only relative. They had no children, and besides being husband and wife, they had been best friends for many years. During the time Bob stayed in the I.C.U., Marcy remained at his side. She never left the hospital for more than an hour at a time. If Bob was going to die, Marcy would be with him.

After about a month passed, it began to seem that maybe Bob was not going to die. He had been weaned from the ventilator and somehow his kidneys had started to make urine. The tube feedings and hyperalimentation began to restore his strength, and the antibiotics had gotten the infections under control. Judy was both happy and sad when Bob was moved to the step-down unit.

But, he looked terrible. Although he moved all his extremities and opened his eyes when spoken to, he remained extremely restless and did not follow any commands. He had to be turned in the bed and lifted into the chair. He was incontinent. Now it was time to transfer him to a rehabilitation center to try to help him improve. But Marcy refused. She wanted to take Bob home. She would take care of him, she told the staff. Judy did not try to talk Marcy out of this; she knew it was what Marcy had to do.

After nine weeks in the hospital, Marcy signed Bob out against medical advice and the volunteer ambulance squad helped her take Bob home. When Judy called the house from time to time to check on Bob, Marcy simply said Bob was making some progress. After a while, Judy stopped calling and they lost touch.

A year later, Judy left the surgical intensive care unit and joined the staff of the radiology nursing department. This particular day, Judy was working in the CT scanning area and went into the scanning room to interview the next out-patient to see which type of intravenous contrast she would administer. The history on the requisition simply said that the patient was having a CT scan of the abdomen as a follow-up to surgery.

The patient was just coming into the room, dressed in a hospital gown. He was big and strong and handsome and had a warm smile on his face. Judy introduced herself and he shook her hand firmly. When she asked the patient what type of surgery he had had, he said, "Well, I sure don't remember any of this, but they tell me my aorta blew right here on this table. That was a few years and eighty-five pounds ago."

And suddenly Judy knew who this was! Her eyes filled with tears as she looked at the miracle in front of her. "Bob," Judy said softly. He reached out and hugged her, but it was obvious that he didn't recognize her. "Marcy's outside," he said.

Judy turned and walked away from Bob, out to the lady who had helped make this miracle happen. They looked at each other and the memories of those times so long ago came back. "Judy," Marcy said. "You were the only one who believed that I could do this. I thought of you often when things got rough. And look at him now."

Yes, Judy thought, as she started to laugh. Just look at him now.

THE GIFT

He had been feeling very tired lately. When he came home from work, he just flopped on the couch and stayed there. He didn't feel like playing with his kids either. He just had no energy to do anything. There were a lot of other vague symptoms. He had no appetite any more. In fact, much of the time he was a bit nauseated. He just didn't feel right. John knew something was wrong.

Lorraine, John's wife, was a nurse with years of experience. It might have been her imagination, Lorraine thought, but John's color looked different. He looked almost a bit sunburned. But this was the middle of the winter and John never spent any time outside. Could he be jaundiced?

Finally, Lorraine convinced John that he needed to see a doctor, and after extensive testing, he was diagnosed with hepatitis C and liver failure. He was put under the care of liver specialists but within two months, John had deteriorated rapidly. His liver function was failing. John, a 33 year old husband and father of three, needed a liver transplant to survive.

And that began the ordeal which was to last almost a year. John was worked up completely to see if he was a candidate for a transplant. By the time he was put on the list, it seemed like a lifetime. But, finally he got that beeper, and the wait began. John was A positive, a common blood type. That seemed to put things in his favor. Surely, someone who was A positive would die and the family would be willing to donate organs? Right?

Well, John and Lorraine saw that it really wasn't that simple. First of all, they both felt like ghouls. When they thought about it, they couldn't believe that they were actually hoping somebody would die. But that's the way it was for them and probably for all patients waiting for organs. They found themselves turning to look at each other whenever they heard a police siren. If they were out in the car and saw a flashing red light, they felt the adrenalin rise as they realized they were hoping there was an accident.

Lorraine, being an I.C.U. nurse, was in a difficult position. If a patient was admitted with anything that might prove fatal, Lorraine started looking up his or her blood type. It got so that she refused to take care of anybody who wasn't more than a routine surgical or medical patient. She didn't want to take care of someone who might be an organ donor. What if she really wanted her patient to die so that her husband could live? She found going to work so stressful that it was hard for her to walk through those unit doors every day, not knowing what she was going to find.

Lorraine knew that John's liver could come from anywhere in the state, and, in certain instances, anywhere in the country. But the day that Lorraine arrived at work and found the people there from the transplant network was the day that Lorraine wasn't sure she could continue to work as a critical care nurse. In that case, the patient was not John's blood type and, in fact, he turned out not to be a suitable organ donor. But that was the turning point for Lorraine. She had to work to support them, but it was hard.

All this time John had been in and out of the hospital, the transplant center in which he was a patient. Due to the fact that his liver now had minimal function, John had to regularly receive blood products and medication to keep him stabilized as he waited for the call that might never come in time. John had three "false alarms," times when his beeper went off to tell him a potential donor had been found. Between the emotional and the physical burdens, these times really took their toll. During the third and final false alarm, John had been admitted and prepped, only to learn that the donor liver was not suitable after all. It was very tough.

Then one night the call came for real. They had found a new liver for John. The surgery itself turned out to be technically very difficult, and it took more than sixteen hours. Within a few days, the first of many complications set in. From rejection to bone marrow failure, John went through three months of hell. Many liver recipients are discharged home within a few weeks. Not John. In fact, it was doubtful that John would ever live long enough to even go home again.

But through it all, John and Lorraine stayed together. They lived one day at a time, and then those days turned into weeks and the weeks turned into months. And, slowly but surely, John began to recover. Today John is not yet physically able to return to the work he used to do. But, he is active and happy and feels like a new person. John and Lorraine speak often at organ awareness functions and John is active in support groups to help other patients waiting for organs. With each day that passes, John and Lorraine give thanks for their new life. And they thank the family who, by their donation, so generously gave John the gift of life.

YA GOTTA BELIEVE

They called her "The Fire Engine Kid." She had been driving down the street on a beautiful summer day with her car windows closed, the air conditioning on, and the radio blasting. She never heard the sirens. As she turned the corner, the fire engine hit her head on. Kristen went right through the windshield.

For three weeks she lay in a coma, and it looked as if she was going to die. The fireman came to visit every day. This kid was only seventeen years old, just starting to live. Even though the accident was nobody's fault, the fireman felt horrible, They had kids her age.

Then, one day Kristen began to move her arm and respond to pain. She started to wake up. Among other injuries, Kristen's jaw had been shattered. Her teeth had been wired together and she breathed through a tracheostomy. And, she had bled inside her head. But, she was getting better.

Many months of recovery and rehabilitation lay ahead for Kristen. It took a lot of tender loving care and patience, because as with all people who are severely head injured, there are bad days mixed with the good ones. Kristen needed little things to make her feel special. everyone pitched in. One of the nurses laughingly remembers the day she decided to give Kristen a bubble bath and almost drowned her in the tub, remembering just before she lay her back in the water that she had a tracheostomy which would suck in the soapy water. Whoops! Kristen laughed too. Later.

Anyway, Kristen got better, and was discharged. Months later she came walking back in to visit all the nurses who took care of her and watched her slowly bur steadily improve. She was one of their miracles. See, miracles happen, and they happen more often than people realize. Any nurse who has been around for awhile will remember his or her own Kristen. Patients who never were supposed to live but who beat the odds. There are numerous families who were given dire predictions concerning their loved ones, only to have them home once again, happy and healthy.

There was a young man who, on the hundredth day of his coma, began to move his hand and flicker his eyes. The next day, his family brought in a big cake for the staff with these words spelled out in the icing:

"100 Days -- Ya Gotta Believe"

Why do these things happen? Why does one patient who has been given no chance of survival wake up and walk out of the hospital, while others die or remain hopelessly brain damaged? Do we know? Will we ever know? Or maybe, more importantly, should we know? The Kristens of this world show us just how much we don't understand, and how little control we really have. Sometimes, ya really just gotta believe!

SECTION TWO

EXPECT THE UNEXPECTED

MURPHY'S LAWS: THE HOSPITAL VERSION

1. Visitors always approach the desk just when both shifts are seated for report and it looks like there's a big coffee break in progress.

2. Surgeons never make rounds when their patients are sitting up in a chair, taking deep breaths, and using their incentive spirometers. They always arrive when their patients are crumpled up at the bottom of the bed.

3. "D/C IV" orders are always given just after you've changed all your I.V. and piggyback tubings.

4. Technologists arrive to do portable x-rays only after the patients have been turned and positioned perfectly on their sides.

5. If there is ever a dinner tray mix-up, it is always the NPO patient who gets (and eats) a full regular meal.

6. Radiology, nuclear medicine, ultrasound, and CT departments only call for patients just after they have been placed back in their beds.

7. Patients ask for pain medications immediately after the order has been D/C'd because you have assured the doctor that they no longer have pain.

8. Discharge orders are written only after the patient's bed has been changed for the day.

9. Oncoming shift nurses call in sick only on the days when you are trying to leave early.

"Murphy's Laws: The Hospital Version," by Linda Strangio, RN, MA, CCRN is reprinted with permission of *The Nursing Spectrum,* New York/New Jersey Metro Edition, Vol. 3, No. 6, March 11, 1991.

COFFEE TIME

It was a very busy day, and nobody had time to go to break. Sue walked out of the pantry with the patient's overstuffed chart tucked under her arm. Besides the chart, she had three Styrofoam cups of coffee balanced precariously between her hands. "Oh, Jane and Jim," Sue called out to the other nurses, "Let's stop for a few minutes and have some coffee." At that precise moment, Sue stumbled and all three coffee cups went flying, as did the big fat chart. When everything hit the floor, almost all the pages in the three week old chart were soaked with coffee.

Without a second thought, Sue grabbed a stretcher and spread out all the sheets on it to dry. Now as luck would have it, the patient's attending physician (who was not exactly known for his sense of humor) picked that exact minute to make rounds. Into the nurses' station he strode, and without looking up, demanded his patient's chart. "Duhh," cleverly replied Sue. "Which part of it would you like?" With that Sue burst into hysterical laughter. The doctor looked at her, looked at the stretcher with its wet coffee-smelling pages, shook his head and walked out of the unit without saying a word.

Sue, still laughing wildly, went back into the pantry for more coffee. By this time everyone else was laughing too. Now it really was break time.

SOUNDS OF NURSES

1. "Open your mouth. Here. Close your mouth. Swallow this pill. Swallow. Swallow. Swallow. Is it down? Let me see. Open your mouth. Stick out your tongue. Close your mouth. Swallow. Swallow."

2. "We're going to lift you from your bed to this chair. No, no. Let go of the side rail. You won't fall."

3. "No, you can't get back in bed just yet. You've only been up in the chair for five minutes. It's good for you to stay up for a while."

4. "Try to stay on your side. No, don't turn back. That's why this pillow is here. Lean back against it. No, no, don't turn back."

5. "I'm going to take your blood pressure. No, it was four hours ago, even though it probably does seem like only 10 minutes ago."

6. "You're still cold? You have 4 blankets on you. O.K. I'll find another blanket.

7. "I know you don't like needles. Nobody likes needles. But you have to have some more blood drawn. Let the lady draw your blood. I'll stay and hold your hand."

8. "You have a tube in your bladder. That's why you feel like you have to go. No, you won't wet the bed. It's O.K. Just let the urine go. It's coming out through the tube.

9. "You need something for pain. You need to take these shots. You just had a big operation. We don't want you to be in pain. No, you won't become a

drug addict from these pain shots."

10. "I know you feel a little bit scared. Let me sit with you for a few minutes. I'll do some of my paper work here while you fall asleep. Will that help you?"

11. "It's O.K. to feel angry. You're sick of being sick. You want to go home and be with your family and sleep in your own bed. You don't want to go through this any more."

12. "It's O.K. to cry."

PIZZA

It was the end of the season and their bowling team had just clinched first place. Even though it was late and they all had to be at work early the next morning, the team decided to go out for pizza and celebrate their win.

So off they went to the local pizzeria. There were five of the them on the team, and like all teams in this hospital league, they sure were a mixed up crew. There was a physician, a carpenter, a social worker, a secretary, and a nurse. This team had been together for four years now, and as different as they were, they were very much alike. They really had fun and enjoyed being together.

Well, the pizza came and they all started eating. Peg, the nurse, was having a ball and laughing out loud. As usual, she was talking and eating at the same time. Now, probably because she had so much to say, she just didn't feel like wasting time doing something as unimportant as chewing her food before she swallowed it. So Peg took a big bite of the pizza, followed by a huge swallow. The last thing Peg remembered was the sharp pain as the food went down. "Ow," she said, and that was it. A few seconds later, Peg's eyes rolled back in her head and she started to convulse.

Now, Peg was not awake to know any of what followed, but she sure heard about it later. That poor bowling team! One of them almost fainted herself when she saw what happened to Peg. And as for the doctor amongst them, Dr. Ted couldn't believe what he was seeing. Of course everyone started yelling at him to do something, and as is only natural, he was literally frozen in his seat for a few seconds. Then all the people in the pizza place, which naturally was packed, got crazy and started yelling to call 911 and grabbing at Peg to do their own versions of CPR. All this, of course, made everything worse since Peg had a strong pulse and, after her seizure was over, began breathing very nicely on her own. Peg obviously didn't need CPR and poor Dr. Ted had to use all his energies to push people away and keep them from breaking Peg's ribs or smashing some of her vital organs.

By the time the ambulance arrived, Peg was wide awake and had no idea what had happened to her. She found herself lying on the floor, surrounded by her panicky bowling teammates who were, by this time, trying to keep her from getting up and running out the door. To say she was mortified is an understatement.

So Peg was admitted to her own hospital and put on her own telemetry floor. And, her friend, Dr. Ted, became her own admitting physician that night, once he recovered from the shock of seeing his buddy turn blue in front of his eyes. The first thing Peg asked, by the way, was if she had been incontinent, because if she was, she told them, she was quitting not only the bowling team, but her job and nobody would ever see her again. No, they told her, she was not incontinent. The only thing she lost that night was her dignity. Oh, and maybe a little mucus when she had her seizure. But that was no big deal.

Well, Peg was worked up for an irregular heartbeat and a seizure disorder and everything else people who pass out and have seizures are worked up for. And, as expected, everything was totally negative. The episode was blamed on swallowing a giant clump of unchewed pizza and having it dig into some nerve or something on the way down. Maybe it wasn't worded exactly that way but that's what it meant, all right.

Two days later, Peg was discharged and she came back to work the following Monday. Peg swore she would never eat a slice of pizza again, but everyone knew she was lying.

And at the bowling banquet that next month, when everyone was sitting and enjoying their delicious meals, a specially prepared pizza was brought to Peg's table. It was a special gift from her bowling team to thank Peg for their unforgettable evening that night in the pizza place.

MORE OF MURPHY'S LAWS

1. If your district has five discharges, you will be doing five admission assessments and ten pages of orders before your shift is over.

2. Codes are called only on the busiest of days and only when you are the most short staffed.

3. If you even <u>think</u> to yourself that you're going to have a quiet shift, everything goes wild.

4. Doctors always call about or come to see their patients the minute their nurses go to break.

5. Doctors arrive to do procedures just as the nurse is trying to reach the cafeteria before it closes.

6. Patients have to go to the bathroom the moment they are settled in their wheelchairs to go to physical therapy.

7. Patients with the worst veins are the ones who manage to pull out their IV's.

8. The STAT floor stock medication you have to give is never in stock.

9. The one day you are finally well staffed is the day someone gets pulled.

"More of Murphy's Laws," by Linda Strangio, RN, MA, CCRN as reprinted with permission of *The Nursing Spectrum*, New York/New Jersey Metro Edition, Vol. 3, No. 9, April 12, 1991.

A LITTLE FRESH AIR

It was 2 o'clock in the morning. Mr. McKinley's cardiac alarm had been sounding all night because he was mildly confused and he kept tugging on his monitor wires. Marie walked down the hall with a couple of new leads in her hands, intending to find a way to attach them high on his shoulders where he would have a harder time reaching them. The bed was empty. Mr. McKinley was gone, his three IV bags attached to their hooks but draining fluids onto the floor. His hand restraints were tied to the bed. Marie ran into the next room and then the next and then up and down the hall. Gone.

Yelling for someone to call Security, she checked the utility rooms and the medication room. Empty. She knew he couldn't have gotten out of the unit through the main doors since there were people in the nurses' station, so the only way was out the back emergency door. She ran down the stairs, finding it hard to imagine that he would have enough strength to get that far. After all, only two days earlier he had had a long abdominal surgical procedure and had multiple drains and tubes in him. But Mr. McKinley was gone.

Security was checking the building when the call came from the city police department. A lady two blocks away had called them to say that there was a naked man in her yard throwing stones against the side of the house. It was, of course, Mr. McKinley.

About twenty minutes later he was wheeled back into the unit covered with a blanket. His foley, N/G tube, and all his dressings were gone and there were dirty leaves clinging to the staples of his dripping operative incision. One remaining penrose drain was sticking out of his abdomen, and his feet and legs were covered with blood-spattered mud.

"Mr. McKinley," moaned Marie. "What did you do?"

"I went for a walk," cheerily reported Mr. McKinley. "I needed the exercise."

Mr. McKinley did fine and was discharged after a week. The walk seemed to do him a lot of good.

BOWLING NIGHT

It was time for her to leave for the day. As she left to punch out at the radiology time clock, Linda noticed the old lady on the stretcher in the waiting area. On her way back to get her coat, she took a longer look. The lady had just been sent over from the emergency department for a CT scan of her brain, and she was probably more than ninety years old.

Uh, oh, thought Linda to herself. This patient looks bad. In fact, she has code potential. The lady's head was bent over and her eyes were rolled back in her head. Her respirations were very shallow. Linda went inside the scanning room and found the other radiology nurse. "You'd better do that lady next," she said to Eileen. "Then get her back to the ER right away."

Linda was zipping up her jacket when the secretary from the CAT Scan office ran in. "Someone better come out and look at this patient," she said. "She doesn't look so good." Eileen and one of the technologists ran out through the door. Two seconds later the tech ran back in, yelling at Linda to come help Eileen. Cursing to herself, Linda threw her pocketbook on the desk, and pulling her jacket off, she ran outside. The lady was in the process of taking her last breath. "Should we call a code?" asked Eileen.

Well, they say that life flashes before your eyes at certain times. In this case, an entire scenario went through Linda's mind in a matter of two seconds. They had a code in the radiology department three days earlier, and that also was just before it was time to leave. It had taken Linda an extra hour to stay and restock the crash cart and do all the paper work and make all the phone calls. The very same thing was going to happen again now, and tonight was her bowling night in the hospital bowling league. Bowling started in less than one hour and she still had to go home and change before leaving for the bowling alley. She had the lowest average in the entire league and if she wasn't there, they would have to deduct ten points off her average and her teammates would kill her.

On the other hand, the emergency department was on this floor, just a few corridors away. If they could race this lady back to the ER before she really and truly stopped breathing for good, they could code her there. After all, that's where she really belonged. And a code in the ER is no big deal. They code people all day long in the emergency room. She was too sick to have been left out in this hall all alone anyway, not even on a monitor or anything.

"Should we call the code?" again asked Eileen after this two second eternity. "No," answered Linda, making her great decision. "We're taking her back to the ER! Come on, Eileen. Let's go!"

So off they went, the two maniac nurses and the poor dying patient. But as luck would have it, the stretcher which this lady had been put on was probably the oldest stretcher in the hospital. It was also, no doubt, the heaviest, most bulky, and the most off-balanced. Each wheel moved in its own direction, with none of them synchronized so that the stretcher could go in a straight line. So when they attempted to go forward, the stretcher instead moved in little jerks, first to the left and then to the right and then in short turning motions.

The faster they attempted to go, the wilder the stretcher's movements got. The lady still had a pulse, but Linda and Eileen knew that after about two more minutes of not breathing, the pulse was going to disappear. As they attempted to run with the stretcher, they narrowly missed banging into several people who were simply walking in the hall.

"Hurry! Run!" The words were repeated over and over as Linda and Eileen frantically worked their way to the emergency room with the wayward stretcher. But they could neither hurry nor run, since this worn out stretcher with the rusted wheels obviously had a mind of its own. It seemed to both of the nurses that they were moving in slow motion. As they rounded the last corner before the entrance to the emergency department, the stretcher broke loose and crashed into the big fire doors. The heavy doors slammed closed right on the stretcher, bouncing the poor lady up into the air and then down again. Somehow the big bump must have opened the patient's airway, because as her head flew up she took a big gasping breath and her eyes slowly opened.

Then by some miracle, they suddenly found themselves with the patient in front of the main nurses' station of the emergency department. "Uh, excuse me," said Linda, trying to appear calm and controlled so that the ER staff would never know that they had raced her back to the emergency room just so they wouldn't have to open the radiology crash cart. "This lady looks like she is going to code so we brought her back from CAT Scan."

"Oh, don't worry about that," pleasantly answered the ER nurse without even looking up. "She came in from a nursing home and she's a definite D.N.R. I guess someone forgot to tell you. Sorry. Just put her in the holding area."

Eileen and Linda brought the lady into the rear of the holding area and parked the rickety old stretcher against the wall. The little old lady, by this time, was breathing nicely on her own and her pulse was strong. It seemed that they had invented a new type of CPR, which worked by flying people up into the air and down again. Slowly and quietly they walked back to the CT department. They didn't even look at each other.

That night at the bowling alley, Linda bowled the three worst games of her entire life. The team dropped down into last place, and everyone really did hate her. God paid her back, but good.

STILL MORE OF MURPHY'S LAWS

1. As soon as you tell the oncoming shift that you have taken the restraints off your patient because she is now perfectly alert and oriented, she pulls out her tubes and falls out of bed.

2. The chart that the attending physician can't find is always right there in the rack.

3. Both you and your patient get tube feeding baths whenever you are absolutely positive you can unclog the plugged feeding tube.

4. The more you rush to hang an IV, the surer you are to poke a hole in the bag with the IV spike.

5. Foley bags you try to empty in the dark, so as not to waken your patient, end up being emptied directly into your shoe.

6. The fresh post-op patient, to whom you have been sneaking tiny amounts of ice chips, tells the surgeon that the "nice nurse" has been giving her lots of ice water.

7. The days when you liberally sprinkle talcum powder over the patient's draw sheet is the day that the physician (in a dark blue suit) decides to sit on the bed to have a long talk with the patient.

8. The chart that falls completely apart when you drop it is the one belonging to a patient who has been on your unit for a minimum of one month.

"Still More of Murphy's Laws," by Linda Strangio, RN, MA, CCRN is reprinted with permission of *The Nursing Spectrum*, New York/New Jersey Metro Edition, Vol. 3, No. 17, August 12, 1991.

BEDLAM

Mr. Richards had developed a severe drug reaction to one or more of his many medications. He had become progressively more confused and was exhibiting bizarre behavior. He was not a candidate for the mental health unit, because he was quite sick medically. He rambled incoherently most of the time, but yet he could be reoriented if the nurses just stayed and talked to him. Mr. Richards had never attempted to climb out of bed or pull at his tubes, so he was not restrained.

It was four-thirty in the morning. The floor was really quiet and the nurses were at the nurses' station doing their charting, when they heard several thuds and then high pitched whimpering. Elsie and Lousie jumped to their feet, just knowing that something bad had happened. They ran down the hall toward the sound of the noises.

Mr. Richards was standing over his roommate, attempting to choke him. The poor little man he was strangling was flailing his arms ineffectively, trying to breathe. Elsie screamed out loud at what she was seeing, obviously scaring Mr. Richards and causing him to let go of the other man. Mr. Richards then bolted from that bed, grabbing hold of an IV pole standing in the hall. In what seemed to be only a split second to Elsie, he picked up the pole and ran over to Anthony, an eighteen year old boy who was in a coma from head injuries suffered in a car accident. Mr. Richards cracked Anthony over the head with that pole and then began running up and down the unit, smashing windows and glass panels as he ran.

By this time, the other nurses were in the middle of the unit, absolutely terrified. Someone ran to the phone and called a cardiac arrest code, deciding that was the fastest way to get the most help. Before anyone could arrive, though, Mr. Richards smashed one of the exterior windows with his trusty IV pole, climbed out on the ledge, and jumped. He landed on the roof two stories below, breaking both legs.

All this happened within a five minute period. Most of the patients in the unit slept right through all the action, totally unaware of the bedlam around them. It took quite a while to calm the staff down, however. As the word spread throughout the hospital, people seemed to arrive from everywhere. Elsie and Louise were more than just a little upset.

The little man that Mr. Richards tried to strangle was OK except for being scared to death. The eighteen year old boy went for emergency skull x-rays and a CT scan, which showed no new injuries. However, a few hours later, morning arrived and Anthony's parents came walking in to visit, carrying a box of Dunkin

Donuts for the nurses. They walked in on a resident sewing up the gash on Anthony's head as the maintenance men were boarding up the window next to his bed. A very reassuring scene.

Mr. Richards was admitted to the intensive care unit for treatment of multiple injuries. A few days later he was totally lucid and had absolutely no memory of what had happened.

IT'S ONLY GAS PAINS

Her stomach had been hurting for a while, maybe a few weeks or so, and it was only a little bit bloody the first time she vomited. It was nothing to get very excited about and she kept on taking the Mylanta.

Later that night when she was alone watching television, she vomited again. This time she really got scared. It was bright red and there seemed to be a lot of blood. Rose called her husband and then her doctor, who happened to be an obstetrician. You see, Rose was seven and a half months pregnant.

By the time she hung up the phone, Rose felt like throwing up again. But this time she never made it to the bathroom. Within one minute she had vomited mouthfuls of blood and clots all over the living room sofa. She had just enough strength to dial 911 before she passed out.

When Rose came to, she was in the emergency room of the hospital and somebody was stuffing a long tube down her nose into her stomach. She was gagging and retching and vomiting blood all around the tube.

And that began Rose Campos and her unborn baby's stay in the intensive care unit. The initial endoscopy showed a huge and actively bleeding gastric ulcer which was vigorously treated medically. Nobody in their right mind wanted to put a seven and a half month pregnant woman through any type of operation, let alone a serious one as that would surely be.

So for the next two weeks Rose stayed in the I.C.U. bed with a fetal monitor on her belly. She received a total of twelve units of blood and lots of fresh frozen plasma. Her nasogastric tube continued to have bouts of bloody drainage and she received lots of medications to try to heal the ulcer. The ultrasounds showed a healthy baby, but one small enough to need more time inside his mother.

Rose had constant abdominal pain and she became very restless. In an attempt to sedate her and keep her labor from starting, she was put on a morphine drip. She looked terrible. Her color was ashen and she moaned all the time. Rose's husband kept a vigil at her bedside, staring from her to the fetal monitor which was watching his unborn baby.

At one point, they had to stop the morphine because Rose stopped responding to the nursing staff and they were afraid they were going to lose both her and the baby. Then one night after more than two weeks in the I.C.U., Rose suddenly sat up in her bed and began to have projectile vomiting right around her tube. Thick red blood clots came right from her mouth, hitting the curtain around her bed.

That was it. There was no more waiting. Rose was rushed to the operating room that night, where surgeons removed almost her entire stomach. She received eight more pints of blood, and then stabilized. She made it through the surgery and so did the baby. Everything looked good. She probably would recover nicely and hopefully would make it through the full term pregnancy.

That was the idea until Rose's fourth post-op day when she once again began to complain of abdominal pain. "It's just gas, Rose," Marilou told her. "Everyone has gas when their intestines are just starting up again. Nothing to worry about." Yeah, right, Marilou.

So Rose's "gas" pains got worse and the Demerol just wasn't helping her anymore. A normal post-operative patient would ambulate to move the gas along, but remember Rose wasn't a normal post-op patient. She was being kept on bedrest to keep her from going into labor. The baby wasn't ready yet.

Well, apparently that baby didn't go along with what everyone else wanted, because he was just about ready to come out. When the obstetrician arrived a few minutes later, he somehow figured out that Rose looked a little different than a person who has gas. His examination showed that Rose was fully dilated and ready to deliver. "Get her to the delivery room!" he yelled as he took off up the stairs to the third floor.

"Oh my God, Rose," screamed Marilou. "Don't do this to me! Please don't have this baby! Hold it in!" Marilou continued to babble these reassurances to Rose as she dragged the heavy bed out of the room by herself, pulling all her equipment with her. Her friend Zenda grabbed the foot of the bed and together they ran for the elevator. Zenda laughed hysterically the whole time while Marilou continued to plead with Rose to hold the baby in.

Once they got on the elevator, Marilou started saying crazy things out loud like, "Oh, what if this elevator gets stuck, or what if the wheel falls off the bed and it won't roll any more?" Rose just kept moaning and screaming and Zenda just kept on laughing and laughing.

They finally got off at the third floor, and when they did they realized they had absolutely no idea which way to go. Neither of them had ever set foot in the obstetrical department and didn't even know which building it was in, just that it was on the third floor somewhere. They stopped and looked at each other and Marilou suddenly screamed out loud, "Help! Help!" Rose was rolling around in the bed and Zenda was doubled over laughing.

Suddenly, as if from nowhere, two OB nurses appeared in their blue scrubs. They didn't have to ask if this was the patient. They saw two loony I.C.U. nurses in their pink scrubs and they just knew. They took the bed and without a word they rolled it down the hall, around the corner, and through the doors into the birthing center. Marilou and Zenda, who were worried only about themselves by this time and certainly not about Rose, were saved by the two blue angels.

Anyway, it turned out that Rose had a normal vaginal delivery about two minutes after she arrived in the delivery room. The baby came into this world awake and crying and in great shape. He was just under five pounds and was in perfect health.

Rose, being now a post-partum as well as a post-operative patient, had a super recovery and went home five days after the birth. Two years later she began to work at the hospital in one of the business offices, and she and Marilou became friends. Rose and her teeny weeny little stomach eat lunch together with Marilou all the time now and they still talk about that crazy night, when the stork won out over the I.C.U. nurses.

MURPHY'S LAWS: PART FOUR

1. Febrile patients break their temps in drenching sweats only after you have finished completely changing all their linen.

2. The doctor cuts the KCL in the IV to 20 meq only seconds after you have just mixed your 1000cc bag with 40 meq.

3. Blood tubes that break or get "lost" contain blood from patients who needed three people to find the vein.

4. As soon as you tell a family that a patient is much better, feels very comfortable, and has a good appetite, the patient tells the same family that she is in terrible pain, can't eat, can't sleep, and feels like she is going to die.

5. The day that you get only half your linen delivery is the day that half of the patients on your floor are incontinent.

6. IV tubings pop off their needles and soak you when you just brush against them, but when you try to loosen tubings to change them they seem to be held in cement.

"Murphy's Laws: Part Four," by Linda Strangio, RN, MA, CCRN is reprinted with permission of *The Nursing Spectrum*, New York/New Jersey Metro Edition, Vol. 4, No. 23, November 2, 1993.

THE LIFESAVER

The surgery had gone fairly well and Mr. Lopez was back from the recovery room. Barbara had medicated him for pain, and now Mr. Lopez was sleeping peacefully.

Dr. Walters was the only physician involved with the care of this patient, since Dr. Walters trusted nobody but himself. He never called consults or allowed residents to go near his patients. Besides being a general surgeon, he considered himself a specialist in everything. He could manage respiratory failure, heart disease and renal insufficiency. He knew everything about infection control and was up on all the latest antibiotic use. Whether it was a low protein or a high potassium, Dr. Walters could deal with it. When a patient needed to be intubated, Dr. Walters was the expert who managed that ventilator. There was nobody who came to close to him, and so he wanted nobody's help. He made all of this perfectly obvious, and so his medical staff colleagues barely tolerated him. He was a decent surgeon, though, and you couldn't take that away from him.

Needless to say, the nurses couldn't stand this man, and he did not exactly relate well to them. Nurses could do nothing right, and they were simply there to empty bedpans and follow his orders. After all, he was the boss, wasn't he? Yukk.

So on this particular evening Mr. Lopez had been pretty stable for about six hours and everyone expected an uneventful night with him. He was just a routine post-operative patient.

Barbara glanced into Mr. Lopez' room as she walked back down the hall to the medication room and something caught her eye. She thought she saw something red on top of the thermal blanket. She entered the room and as she got closer to the bed she realized that there was nothing on top of the blanket, but instead the entire lower half of the blanket was red. Blood red.

Barbara whipped back the blanket and saw that Mr. Lopez was lying in a pool of blood and clots, a puddle which reached from his waist down almost to his ankles. His dressing was so soaked with blood that it was not adhering to the skin anymore. She pulled off the sopping wet pile of gauze and saw the red blood just pouring out from between the staples of the surgical incision. Mr. Lopez was close to bleeding to death.

Grabbing a pile of fresh dressings, Barbara put pressure over the bleeding abdominal wound. She had no idea if the blood was coming from a vessel close to the surface or something deep in the abdomen, but she couldn't stand there and do nothing. At least there was a chance that whatever pressure she put over the area might help to stem the blood loss.

While she stood there with Mr. Lopez, one of the other nurses put out a call to Dr. Walters. There was no question as to whether or not he was on call that night, since the great Dr. Walters never signed out to a covering surgeon. Nobody was good enough, in his opinion, to cover his patients. He took call every night of his life. It was bad enough that he was forced to have another surgeon assist him in the operating room with his major cases.

Beth came in to see what she could do to help out. Barbara gave her job of holding pressure over the incision while she ran out to get equipment to start another IV line. She got a second line going and opened both rates so that the IV fluids would run as fast as possible. By this time, Mr. Lopez' blood pressure was only ninety over sixty and his pulse rate was climbing. Barbara put the head of the bed down low and called the lab to get him typed and crossed-matched for another six units of blood. Then there was nothing else to do except keep reassuring Mr. Lopez that he would be fine and to wait for Dr. Walters to return the phone call.

After what seemed like an eternity, the phone call came and it was just as Barbara expected. "What do you want?" Dr. Walters asked nastily. "This had better be something important. You are disturbing my dinner." When Barbara explained what had happened, he simply responded, "OK, and then slammed the phone on her.

"I hate this man," announced Barbara. She went back into Mr. Lopez' room to relieve Beth with the blood soaked dressings. Then they waited. They purposely did not attempt to change the sheets since they knew without a doubt that Dr. Walters would never believe their description of what had happened. He had to see it.

Within ten minutes Dr. Walters strode into the room. He threw off the covers, giving the panicky Mr. Lopez a full view of everything that had leaked out of his body. He pulled Barbara's hand off the dressings and ripped them off of the wound. Again he simply said "OK" and walked out of the room.

Beth followed him to the phone and listened to him yell at the OR nurses, giving them orders and screaming at them to be ready for his patient within two minutes. He then came back to the bedside and barked at Barbara, "Get him to the OR." Then he turned and walked out of the unit. That was it. He said nothing to the patient, who by this time was absolutely terrified.

The nurses tried to calm Mr. Lopez down, and even attempted to joke with him. They took him, right in his bed, to the operating room where the staff was ready and waiting for him. Barbara told the operating room nurses and the anesthesiologist what she had done in regard to the blood work and the IV fluids. Knowing that Dr. Walters would never think to call the family, Barbara did just that. She called his wife, explaining that Mr. Lopez was back in the operating room because he had some bleeding from his wound. He would be fine, she said, but maybe Mrs. Lopez needed to come to the hospital.

Three hours later the recovery room staff called to say that Mr. Lopez was ready to come back, and was awake and stable. He had needed four of the six units of blood and had been given lots of IV fluids, but now it seemed he was stable. And they said that Dr. Walters had spoken to the patient's wife after the surgery.

By the time Mr. Lopez returned to the floor Dr. Walters was long gone, probably back to stuffing his face again. Mrs. Lopez seemed very relieved. She told Barbara that Dr. Walters had saved her husbands life, and that he explained to her how he had found him bleeding to death and he had rushed him back to surgery just in time. What a wonderful man he was, she said. It was as if God himself was right there, in the form of Dr. Walters.

Barbara didn't know if she should laugh or cry. She was just dying to tell this lady just what a pompous ass this guy was, and how the nurses and not the doctor saved her husband. She wanted to blurt out how all this doctor could do was cut and sew and there was more to being a great doctor than that. She almost let go all of her feelings about this nasty self-centered egomaniac who nobody could stand, and how this event was just one of so many which highlighted all the negative characteristics this man constantly manifested. She wanted to tell this lady how everyone in the hospital felt about her precious Dr. Walters.

But she didn't say a word. She just couldn't. Barbara just smiled and said how glad she was that Mr. Lopez was alright now. Then she left the room and went back to the nurses' station to get herself together. The nurses looked at each other and just shook their heads. There was nothing more to be said.

DOCTOR NASTY

It was just another hip repair except for the fact that this lady was ninety-three years old and weighed only seventy-eight pounds. When she had fallen in the nursing home and broken her hip, she had really lost a lot of blood into the soft tissue of her thigh. It was all swollen and discolored before the surgery and now it really looked terrible.

For someone her size and in her condition, Mrs. MacGregor could really wiggle around in bed. Despite her age, she had gotten around very well before the fall. This woman was used to being independent. She was fully alert and oriented and didn't like to be kept in bed. Her catheter had been removed and she knew she had to ask for a bedpan when she felt she had to go. But knowing what she was supposed to do and doing what she was supposed to do were two different stories.

So Lisa had just returned to the desk and was looking up someone's lab work on the computer when she heard the thud. That familiar sound obviously meant that someone had fallen out of bed. And guess who it was?

Running into Mrs. MacGregor's room, Lisa found exactly what she expected. The little old lady was on the floor, having climbed over the foot of the bed. "Mrs. MacGregor," moaned Lisa. "Where were you going?"

"I had to go to the bathroom, dear," Mrs. MacGregor replied. "I forgot I couldn't walk. I'm just used to doing things on my own. I'm really sorry to have caused you so much trouble."

With one look, Lisa knew this was not going to be just an average fall, one which happens in hospitals all the time. The plastic wedge that had been put between Mrs. MacGregor's legs to keep the new surgery stabilized was loose and her leg was at a weird angle. Lisa sat down on the floor next to her patient and saw that Mrs. MacGregor's left wrist looked funny. First, she had to be lifted back to bed very carefully, because of the tenuous condition of her hip. The last thing they needed to do was cause further damage to the area, so she was rolled like a log and the cardiac arrest board was placed under her pelvis and then lifted up to the bed slowly and carefully.

"Oh, great," said Lisa out loud, suddenly realizing who the orthopedic surgeon was. Of all the orthopods, it had to be this one. When anything out of the ordinary happened with his patients, he routinely carried on like a maniac. And this time was, of course, no exception. According to him, the nurses were idiots, this whole orthopedic unit was a joke, and his patient would have done better if he had sent her directly from the operating room to the casinos in Atlantic City.

Obviously, the hip needed to be x-rayed right away, as did the deformed wrist. By some absolute miracle, when x-ray called up the wet readings of the films, it turned out that the hip was fine. Mrs. MacGregor did, however, have a broken wrist that needed to be casted, and Lisa had to have the pleasure of calling the doctor to tell him the news.

About a half hour later, Dr. Casey strode in through the doors. He was livid. When Lisa had called to give him the x-ray results, he had screamed at her that she was damn lucky that Mrs. MacGregor did not have to go back to the operating room to have her hip redone. "Come in here and help me," he ordered Lisa with controlled fury. "I want to set this wrist and get away from this place and you." Lisa knew Dr. Casey well enough to say nothing. She sedated Mrs. MacGregor and helped Dr. Casey put on the cast. When he finished, he wrote a nasty note in the chart about the patient falling out of bed even though he had specifically written, as he did with all his patients, to keep side rails up.

Gail cursed Dr. Casey as she read the note. The side rails had been up, as they always were with patients like this. He wrote side rail orders only as a legal C.Y.A. (cover your ass) reason, and the note insinuated that the rails were down. She would be sure to write a big fat nurse's note for this one.

An hour later, Mrs. MacGregor started putting on her call light every ten minutes to say she had to go to the bathroom, and every time someone would put her on the bedpan she voided about an ounce. After the sixth time, Lisa checked Mrs. MacGregor's bladder and even though it didn't feel all that distended, Lisa felt sure that it was full.

"Listen up," she said to her buddy Kimberly. "I'm going to stick a catheter in and drain that bladder, and I am not going to call Dr. Casey to ask him if I can do this. No way, no how, will I call that mad maniac and have him scream at me again. I am going to catheterize her and if I find just a little bit of urine in her bladder, it is going to remain our little secret. If I find a big blown up distended bladder, then I will call Dr. Casey and let him know I did something right."

As soon as Lisa put the catheter in she knew that the bladder was full. The urine came pouring out of the tube, and within five minutes Lisa had drained out a quart. The patient, exhausted from the events of the day and from climbing on and off the bedpan every couple of minutes, fell into a deep sleep even before her bladder was totally empty. Finally, she was comfortable. "OK, Kimberly," Lisa announced. "Now I will call the old lunatic and tell him the story which ended well this time."

When Dr. Casey called back, he was very nasty to her. "What have you done now?" he sneered. "Have you overdosed her or maybe caught her other wrist in the side rail or something?"

Lisa took a deep breath. "No, Dr. Casey," she answered. "I wanted to tell you Mrs. MacGregor was voiding in very small amounts. I catheterized her and got a quart of urine and she is much more comfortable now."

"Do you expect congratulations from me?" angrily responded Dr. Casey. "It's your fault in the first place that she couldn't urinate right. After what you put her through, you're lucky she's not dead." And then the bastard hung up.

Lisa wanted to scream right there in the nurses' station. She knew that she could write a letter to the president of the medical staff, telling him how rude and obnoxious this man was. She knew she could make all kinds of scenes, going through her nursing administration right to the president of the hospital. But, she also was fully aware of how powerful this surgeon was and just how many patients and how much money he brought in. And, she knew that Dr. Casey wouldn't even get a slap on the wrist. He would somehow turn this around to make the nurses look incompetent. Also, if she was going to remain in her job, which she was, she was going to have to keep working with him. And there was no question he could make her life miserable if she made waves for him.

So, instead, Lisa wished out loud for him to have a cardiac arrest in the elevator while he was in it all by himself. Then she wished it should get stuck between floors so nobody would even know he was in there. And, by the time they got it moving and found him, it should be many hours later when he was not only dead, but starting to decompose right there on the floor. Oh, and he also should have pooped in his pants just before he died, so he could be found lying in a big smelly mess, preferably by his colleagues.

The picture of this little scene made Lisa feel much better, maybe a little less powerless. And she actually smiled as she sat down to write her nurse's note.

MURPHY'S LAWS FOR THE HOSPITAL: PART FIVE

1. The little old lady who is too weak to feed herself or brush her teeth can still manage to do a sit-up and bring her head right down to her restrained hands to pull out her N/G tube.

2. The attending physician who is much too busy to return your phone call seems to always have time to want you to sit and listen to his jokes when he arrives to make rounds.

3. Missing dentures can usually be found in the laundry (tucked inside a pillow case) or in the dietary department (wrapped neatly in a napkin on a dinner tray).

4. The day you go home with the narcotic keys is the day you've just finished the worst shift you can ever remember.

5. On wild days you manage to get everything done; on the quietest of shifts you forget to change your IV tubings, record your accuchecks, or total your I and O's.

6. The patient who screams when you try to take her blood pressure never makes a sound to warn you that she is pulling out her foley with the balloon fully inflated.

7. Leaky foleys are found only in patients who need three or more nurses to change their beds.

THE IMPATIENT PATIENT

It was Christmas week, the time when no nurse who really cares about her co-workers wants to call in sick. Staffing is bad enough with people taking extra time off, and the hospital usually works short staffed. So, when Mary Ann started running those fevers, she knew she had to come to work anyway.

The cough wasn't too bad. It was intermittent and dry. The worst part was the pressure in her back. It felt as if she had been punched there, and when she took a deep breath it was hell.

But Mary Ann dragged herself in to work the day after Christmas, and somehow she made it through her shift. She took Tylenol and cough medicine, went home and fell into bed. But the next day, she was worse. She was scheduled to work evenings and she called the unit that morning in tears. She had never felt so horrible, she said. Her mother had been rubbing Ben-Gay on her back but it didn't seem to help. And her temperature was a hundred and two.

Go to a doctor, they told her. You can't keep on like this. But like so many nurses, Mary Ann didn't really have a doctor. Oh, sure, she had all her specialists picked out if she should ever need them, and she was all set if she ever needed brain surgery or went into diabetic coma or anything like that. But there was nobody she could turn to if she just plain got sick.

Sue was one of Mary Ann's best friends and she was there when the call had come in. Sue told Mary Ann that if she was not in the emergency room by three o'clock, she was either going to drive to her house and drag her in, or call an ambulance to go pick her up.

By two o'clock, Mary Ann was on a stretcher in one of the examining rooms. Her blood work had been drawn and a chest x-ray had been taken. As Mary Ann lay on her side breathing little shallow breaths, she heard the voice of her favorite lung specialist saying, "Is she as bad as this chest film looks?" It took Mary Ann a few seconds to realize that Dr. Danning was talking about her.

Mary Ann was admitted to a medical floor with a diagnosis of pneumonia with a pleural effusion. She was started on intravenous antibiotic therapy and nasal oxygen. By this time she had started vomiting, and nobody was sure if this was due to the disease or the medications. Two days later, Mary Ann was no better, and she was transferred to the Concentrated Care Unit.

Dr. Danning decided to do a thoracentesis and drain that pocket of fluid around her lung. Mary Ann was scared to death by this time. She had never been sick in her whole life and now she felt as if she were dying. Her friends sat her up on the side of the bed while Dr. Danning did the tap. Sue talked to her the whole time, telling her that when she got better the unit was going to have a big party for her. Mary Ann cried and vomited through the whole thing, but they got her through it.

As she lay back in the bed, Mary Ann seriously reminded Dr. Danning that the next day was New Years Eve and she just had to work. Nobody, but nobody calls in sick on a holiday, she told him. Dr. Danning looked at her like she was nuts and left the room. Obviously, not being a nurse, he could never understand.

Within a few hours, they had the preliminary report. No wonder she wasn't improving with those antibiotics. Mary Ann had tuberculosis, and she most likely caught it from one of her patients. So she was started on anti-TB. drugs.

Well, New Years Eve came and went and so did New Years Day. Obviously Mary Ann was a patient during that time, not a nurse. And speaking of patients, she was the world's worst. She constantly climbed over her side rails to go to the bathroom because she didn't want any one to know how much diarrhea she was having. Dizzy and nauseated as she was, she barricaded herself in that same bathroom when it came time to get washed because she didn't want to take any kind of chance that someone would see her with her gown pulled down. She never told anyone when her IV was starting to hurt because she didn't want to be stuck again. And so on.

But as they say, the best medicine is a dose of tincture of time, and after about a week, Mary Ann began to get better. And once she started to improve, she continued to do so. After a month in the hospital, Mary Ann was discharged. The day after she went home, she came back to work, telling everyone she had been cleared to do so, but had lost the written medical clearance. Dr. Danning was on vacation, so nobody was able to check with him to find out that she was lying. She did fine and said the best therapy for her was being back to work. Mary Ann continued taking her anti-TB. drugs for a very long time and stayed well. And, as far as anyone knew, nobody ever caught the disease from her.

To this day, when any nurse calls in sick because of the usual cramps, headache, or head cold, people talk about Mary Ann and how she came to work with a chest full of pus. And, nobody can top that.

A BIG MAC ATTACK

There had been some strange people seen wandering through the hospital late at night, away from the patient care areas. Things had disappeared also, like telephones and typewriters. So it was no surprise that some of the people who worked alone in offices were a bit edgy.

The Nursing Administrative offices were lonely at night, and the only activity took place at change of shift when the nursing supervisors gave report. Other than that, the corridor was empty. The only sounds were those of the secretaries' typewriters. And these women were a little scared to be there at night. It was lonely.

So to make the staff feel more comfortable, the nursing administrators decided to close off the department at night by having a window installed through which the night secretaries could speak to whomever came by. Then they could feel more secure behind their locked doors. A great idea everyone thought.

Construction began early one Monday, and by the next day it was just about finished. The wall was up and the window was in. All that it needed was the glass.

Now during the daytime, that same corridor was far from quiet. All the offices were occupied and busy, and the days of the construction were no exception. That afternoon, one of the nursing coordinators, Debbie, decided to run up to the nursing office to pick up her mail. Routine. As she passed by one of the conference rooms, she noticed a meeting in progress with about ten people in attendance. Also routine. She took her mail, chatted a while and then left. Debbie was known to be a bit on the loud side, so she took special pains to keep her voice down when she spoke to people in the hallway. She didn't want to disturb the meeting. It looked important. Besides the nursing administrators, she recognized at least four of the hospital vice-presidents in there.

As Debbie reached the end of the hallway, she suddenly noticed the window. It looked interesting. It reminded her of the drive through window at McDonalds. Goodness knows, she spent enough time there.

The nursing office receptionist was working at a desk inside the room with the new window. She glanced up and waved at Debbie. Suddenly, and obviously without thinking, Debbie walked up to the window and yelled out loud, "Carmela, I want a Big Mac and a chocolate shake." As the words left her mouth, Debbie raised both hands into fists and slammed them down on the window ledge, having absolutely no idea in the world that this was a newly plastered and very soft window.

As soon as her fists hit the window sill, the ledge totally collapsed, smashing downward with globs of wet plaster spurting everywhere. Debbie, her eyes filling with horror at what she had done, just stared at Carmela. Carmela couldn't believe what she had seen. "Oh my God, oh my God," whimpered Debbie. "I didn't know it was wet!" Carmela, unable to speak, simply pointed at the sign above the window. It read in big black letters,

"CAUTION - WET PLASTER"

Debbie looked down at the floor, probably getting ready to faint. Suddenly she saw some of the tools left behind by the workmen. There was a trowel there. Debbie, who had never laid a hand on a trowel or anything remotely similar in her whole life, whispered hoarsely to Carmela, "I'll fix it. Don't tell anyone what I did." She picked up the trowel and swiped it across what was left of the window sill. Big chunks of the plaster pulled loose from the ledge and fell to the floor. It was horrible.

At this point, Debbie panicked. Dropping the trowel, she turned around and ran back down the hall toward the conference room. Opening the door, she burst into the room. The group, engrossed in what they were discussing, looked up at her. "I broke the ledge," she babbled. "I didn't mean to. I was just fooling around, I can't fix it. I'm so sorry. I don't know what to do." And with that Debbie bolted from the room and took off down the hall and out of the department.

Debbie went back to her area and locked herself in the nurses' bathroom. She stayed there a long time, expecting to hear herself paged any minute. She wasn't. She then went back to work and spoke to no one, except when they asked her something. The staff asked her what was wrong, and she told them she didn't feel well. All the time, she waited for the phone to ring, to hear that she was either being fired or committed to the psychiatric unit. But she heard nothing.

Two hours later, Debbie finally got up enough nerve to call Carmela. When Carmela picked up the phone, all Debbie said was, "What happened?" Carmela simply told her that everything was all right, that the workmen had come back and redone the window and cleaned up the mess. And as far as the administrators were concerned, Carmela told her it had all been taken care of. Nobody was going to say a word to Debbie about it.

Debbie knew Carmela had saved her, just the way she always took care of things. Whatever she had told people, they had agreed that nothing good could come of pursuing it. It was over. Temporary insanity or whatever, it was over.

It was several days till Debbie could get up enough courage to go back to the Nursing Administration department again. This time the window glass had been installed and everything looked lovely. Nobody mentioned a thing to her about what happened. But just as she was leaving the department, Fran, one of the secretaries, called to Debbie that she had a message for her. Debbie took the paper and read what was written:

"WOULD YOU LIKE FRIES WITH YOUR ORDER?"

Finally, Debbie could laugh.

EXERCISE

The lady was screaming and yelling non-stop. She was down for a CT scan of her chest, and she was a D.N.R. patient with severe dementia. She also was about five feet tall and weighed bout two hundred and seventy pounds. Judy was the radiology nurse.

"Sarah, lie still," repeatedly yelled Judy, trying to get through to Sarah over the constant screaming. "I have to start this IV to give you the x-ray dye." Well, forget about Sarah lying still. She was wild and thrashing on the table. Somehow, after three tries, Judy finally managed to get the angiocath in the lady whose arms were in perpetual motion. They restrained her in position and then Sarah stopped flailing on the table, although the screaming never stopped.

They talked to Sarah through the microphone during the entire scan, trying to calm her and tell her everything was going well. It was as if they were talking to a stone, because Sarah never heard a word anyone said. She was too busy howling. At the end of the procedure, Judy went in to remove the angiocath. Among the bruises and swelling from other sticks, Judy found an infiltrate of x-ray dye under the skin. Sarah obviously had been pulling the restraints and had dislodged the angiocath.

Oh, great, thought Judy. Not only did she have another statistic for her quality assurance IV infiltration study, but now she had to fight with Sarah to put warm soaks on the area. There was little Judy, barely a hundred pounds, fighting with this two hundred and seventy pound lady who was swinging that swollen arm side to side like a pitcher taking his warm up. "Stop, stop, Sarah," yelled Judy. "I can't hold you. Lie still!" Naturally, Sarah never even slowed down.

"Oh, do you need help?" innocently asked one of the technologists.

"I can't hear you," shrieked Judy. "I'm too busy giving this lady third degree burns. Of course I need help!"

By the time the soak was on, Judy was as wet as the dressing and Sarah's soaking gown. Judy had no way of knowing whether or not the arm was hurting Sarah, since the screaming was at the same level as when she had first rolled off the elevator. And, of course Sarah wouldn't or couldn't answer any questions.

Well, when they finally managed to drag Sarah, screeching at the top of her lungs and once again thrashing wildly, off the scanning table and back on to her stretcher, they noticed a few things. Number one, hidden underneath the strap of the poesy and almost up by her shoulder, was a perfectly good heparin lock, taped securely in place. Judy had never needed to stick her in the first place. And secondly, her name was Anna and not Sarah. Maybe that was one of the reasons they couldn't get through to her. And they also just happened to see that Sarah (or

Anna) had managed to grab hold of her foley catheter and rip it out of her bladder with the balloon fully inflated.

Oh, by the way. The CT scan was perfectly normal.

All in a day's work.

MURPHY'S LAWS FOR THE HOSPITAL: PART SIX

1. Hungry doctors arrive on the floors only minutes after visitors have brought in candies and cakes for the nurses.

2. Other nurses get pulled to your unit only on the quietest shifts so that they believe your floor is the easiest in the hospital and you *never* work as hard as they do.

3. Doctors cannot examine their patients without tearing apart your beautifully made beds.

4. Patients who refuse to eat are the ones who stuff tissues in their mouths, chew their IV tubings in half, and attempt to drink from their urinals.

5. Starving NPO patients are wheeled up to the desk just as you are biting into a juicy jelly donut.

6. Restrained patients always manage to squirm down to the very bottom of the bed or stretcher, just to do it again the minute you pull them up.

7. The patients who are on the most oral medications are the ones who have the hardest times swallowing pills.

8. Patient who have their call bell answered after two minutes tell their families that they were kept waiting forever, while the ones who really have to wait never say a word.

OVERHEAD DEPARTMENT

1.   The old man was out in front of the nurses' station strapped into his gerry chair with a Posey restraint. "Veronica! Veronica! Talk to me!" he screamed over and over again. He wouldn't eat and he wouldn't drink. All he wanted was Veronica. "Mr. Carter," Andrea bargained, "If you drink this big glass of cranberry juice, you can call Veronica on the phone. And that's a promise."

"OK," said Mr. Carter. "Give me the juice." Andrea went to the pantry and returned with a glass of juice. "Here you go," she said, "Now drink up." Mr. Carter took the glass of juice and brought it slowly to his mouth. Then within a split second he turned his head to the side and dumped the cranberry juice all over his ear and down the right half of his face. "Veronica," he yelled into the empty cup. "Where the hell are you? Pick up this phone!"

2.   It was a busy evening in the detox unit. Joe had been pacing up and down the hall for over two hours. Marcia was getting tired just watching him. "Sit down for a while, Joe." Marcia said. Joe walked into the nurses' station and plopped himself down in a chair.

"I'll read this," he announced, grabbing the report clipboard off the desk. "Oh, my," he said to Marcia. "You certainly have a lot of members of the Foley family here in this unit. They must all drink a lot."

3.   Fred was seated in the hall in his wheelchair waiting for the transportation escort to take him to physical therapy. His eyes were squeezed shut. "I can't see! I can't see!" He had been screaming like this all morning. Diana walked by and heard Fred screaming.

"Open you eyes, Fred," she said. Fred did so.

"Oh, my God," Fred screamed. "I can see again. You saved my eyesight, nurse, Oh, thank you. I'll never be able to repay you!"

4.   Jen was sitting at the nurses' station doing her charting and eating a tuna fish sandwich at the same time. There were other people there with her, including an endocrinologist sitting right next to her. The phone rang, and Jen went to pick it up. Somehow, as she said hello, she aspirated the piece of sandwich which was in her mouth right down into her trachea. Jen couldn't speak, but instead she made some kind of weird croaking sound. Dr. Sterry looked up just in time to see her drop the phone and clutch at her throat, in the classic universal choking symbol.

As Dr. Sterry stood up to help her, Jen bolted from her chair and raced into the nurses' bathroom next to the station. Chasing her to the bathroom, he heard the unmistakable sound of the lock clicking shut from the inside. He then heard Jen gagging and trying to cough inside the bathroom as he helplessly pounded on the door. Within a minute, the door opened and Jen emerged. Her face was red and her eyes and nose were red and dripping.

"Are you crazy?" roared Dr. Sterry. "What's wrong with you? You could have died in there!" he screamed at her.

Jen shrugged. "I didn't want you to see me throw up," she explained simply. Dr. Sterry just shook his head and walked away.

PAP SMEARS BY FLASHLIGHT

It had been a terrible day at the hospital. They were short staffed, and as every nurse knows, those are the days that everything goes wrong.

It seemed as if all the patients had to be sent off the floor for different tests and procedures, and little annoying things had happened all day. Medications were not in the bins and they had to be sent for, doctors were unavailable for long periods of time, and the residents seemed to change their orders as fast as the nurses transcribed them. Then to top it all off, the narcotics keys simply disappeared, and after searching everywhere and calling everyone, they turned up on the floor behind the toilet in the nurses' bathroom. Very embarrassing.

So she had left work late, and this was the afternoon that she had been dreading. It was time for her yearly GYN exam. This was not a very big thing to most people, but she hated it. It would be easier to have ten teeth pulled than to go for that PAP smear, she swore. Everyone laughed, but she meant it. How had she gone through three pregnancies and three deliveries, she really didn't know.

It was dusk by the time she got on her way to the doctor's office. She first had rushed home to take a shower and change so she would be nice and clean. It seemed incredible to her that some of the nurses went straight to the gynecologist's office from work. Yukk.

As she drove past the supermarket, she noticed the stream of people coming out. The store was dark and so was the parking lot. There must have been a power failure, she thought. That must have been rough, she smiled, imagining the people waiting on the line with full grocery carts and then not being able to ring the items up at the cash register. She felt sorry for them.

Arriving at the corner, she realized that the traffic lights were also out. Uh, oh, she said to herself. This must be a bigger power outage than just one store. The doctor's office had better not be affected, she thought. She had come this far.

As she pulled up in front of the row of buildings, she realized there were no lights anywhere. A little feeling of uneasiness came over her, but she decided that since it wasn't totally dark yet, the lights inside most likely just don't show up. Wrong.

She walked into the building, which was almost pitch dark. Her doctor's office was on the first floor, and as she opened the door, she saw him sitting on a couch in the waiting room surrounded by a stack of flashlights and talking to his nurse, who had obviously just come in from buying the stuff at the pharmacy next door.

"So. ladies," the doctor said with a laugh to the patients in the waiting room. "It's up to you. Do you want to reschedule or do you want to see if we can get through this?"

She couldn't believe that he could even ask such a question. Of course everyone should reschedule. This was an omen, she felt. She should turn around and go home. She had put off the exam so long anyway that a little more of a wait couldn't hurt. He should just close the office and let everyone leave.

"No, let's go," everyone else in the room said. "Of course we don't want to wait." She was horrified. They must all be nuts or something. This was their chance to escape, and nobody was taking it. She said nothing, since she didn't want to be the only one to jump up and run out. Besides, with her luck and coordination, she'd probably fall down the two front steps of the building in the darkness and make an even bigger scene.

So one by one, the nurse led the ladies into the examining rooms, pointing the way with the flashlight. She just sat there. How could he do a GYN exam in the dark? Not that she exactly liked light. In fact, she always told people that she wished she had a gynecologist who was ninety years old and blind.

When it was her turn, the usher, or rather the nurse, led her into the room. Another flashlight had been turned to face the wall, and when the nurse left, the room was very dim. Hey, she thought. This isn't half bad. It's much more private this way. So she got undressed and sat there wrapped in that gigantic piece of toilet paper they call a gown. At least she didn't feel like she was a lab specimen on display in the bright light.

The doctor came into the room leading the way with the flashlight, so that he didn't fall on his head. He thought the whole thing was funny, since he could barely read the blood pressure in the dark, and he went ahead with the examination in his usual professional and matter-of-fact way. By then he was wearing what she called his coal miner's lamp on his head, but when he was done, she was back in the security of the darkened room. And of course, she was fine and told she was good for another thousand miles. No big deal.

As she wrote out the check for the visit by the light of the flashlight, she thought how weird this had been. Pap smears by flashlight. Hmmn. It was kind of funny. She really should write a story about it.

And she did.

SECTION THREE

RELATIONSHIPS

A PAINFUL STORY

Charlene was a great nurse, everyone thought. She was relatively new at that hospital but the other nurses had quickly gotten to like her. Besides the beautiful nursing care she gave, she always kept her patients comfortable. Why, you could tell that by the amount of pain medication she used. After all, some patients complain of pain at the start of the shift, and when you check to see if they could have a pain shot you find they're way overdue.

Not with Charlene. Her patients got their pain medication every three to four hours. If it was ordered that way, they got it. Charlene worked nights, and her post-op patients were always sleeping peacefully when the day shift came on. And when the oncoming nurse started the narcotic count, she knew right away when Charlene was working; the sign-out sheet was filled right to the bottom of the page.

Charlene worked on a medical-surgical floor, but it was no secret that she much preferred to take care of surgical patients. There was nothing wrong with that of course. Everyone has preferences.

Then some things began to change. Charlene's patients seemed to be more awake and a bit more uncomfortable in the mornings. They told the day nurses that they had received pain shots but the medication didn't help all that much; it kind of just "took the edge off the pain."

This went on for a short while and one day one of the day nurses noticed a couple of weird things. First, Charlene had begun to make a couple of mistakes. For one thing, she had signed out some Demerol to a patient who didn't have any Demerol ordered. When the medication sheet on the patient's chart was checked, there was no mention of any Demerol nor was there any STAT dose ordered on the doctor's order sheet. Then that very same week, there were two patients who had been on Demerol but hadn't needed any pain relief for days. But, on Charlene's shifts, she documented that she had given them pain shots every three hours.

But the final event happened one morning when one of the nurses became suspicious after finding Demerol signed out to a patient who was discharged that day. That same nurse had gotten the Demerol order discontinued two days earlier, since the patient was pain free.

First there was denial. Charlene couldn't possibly be taking narcotics. That doesn't happen with "normal" nurses, nurses just like themselves. How could she be a drug addict and do so much good work? Her attendance was fine and she always looked healthy.

Then came little private whispered conversations. Maybe it was possible after all. They had all noticed little things. Everyone knew she gave a lot of drugs. She always asked for those keys as soon as she got in. And the other night nurses said it was funny that she often told them that their patients had asked her for pain shots. She always volunteered to help out her fellow nurses by medicating their patients. And it was strange that the patients never told their nurses they were hurting.

When it became obvious that something was very wrong, the problem was turned over to the nurse-manager and then to nursing administration. The Board of Nursing was called.

The next few weeks were very traumatic for the nursing staff of that floor. There wasn't one person who didn't really like Charlene as a person or think of her as a good nurse. As the investigation went on, Charlene's co-workers had mixed feelings. There was a lot of anger --- anger at Charlene for several reasons. The nurses felt betrayed by her. How could she trick them like this? How could she cheat and lie and make them go through this charade of assuming everything was normal, while there was a secret investigation going on? And worse, how could she make her patients suffer by taking their drugs and giving them some mild substitute? The whole thing was a rotten mess.

The Board of Nursing wanted some concrete evidence before they confronted her. The nurses knew how important it was to follow the instructions of the authorities, but it was very difficult for them. The next night, two people from the Board of Nursing arrived at the hospital. One of the other night nurses had been asked to watch Charlene and call the nursing office if she noticed anything unusual as far as narcotic administration. At one o'clock, the nurse called down to report that she checked the narcotic sign-out sheet and found that Charlene had already signed out medications for the whole shift, up until six-thirty in the morning.

That was enough. The director of nursing and one of the Board of Nursing members went up to the unit and asked Charlene to take her pocketbook and come down to the nursing office with them. Charlene knew right away what had happened.

It was like opening a floodgate as soon as they began to question Charlene. Her relief at being found out was overwhelming. When asked if they could look in her pocketbook, Charlene quickly dumped it on the table, spilling out four ampules of Demerol and a syringe. She told them that this had been going on for years, and she had become hooked on pain medication after being in a car accident years earlier and spending six weeks in traction.

Charlene also revealed that she had done the same thing before at two other hospitals, but when it was discovered the nursing administration simply asked her to quietly resign. They didn't want any trouble. So Charlene was able to continue doing the same thing again and again. But, in Charlene's own words, she said she "was tired and wanted help and now she could get it."

Charlene's nursing license was taken from her that night, and soon after, the Board of Nursing suspended it. Charlene came up to the unit to clean out her locker, and her former staff members treated her with respect and offered her good wishes and encouragement.

It was what you could call a bittersweet event. When it was all over, only the sadness and compassion was really remembered. There was a lot learned from this, and hopefully, the nurses as well as Charlene would be stronger people because of it.

HAPPY BIRTHDAY

Gerry had been the head nurse of the unit for ten years, and today was her fortieth birthday. She had half expected some kind of a party from her staff, but knew there could be nothing at work.

The Department of Nursing frowned upon that sort of thing, since recently there had been several complaints from families about unprofessional nursing behavior. Gerry wasn't exactly sure what that meant, but she and all the other head nurses had been told to always maintain quiet and decorum on their floors. Gerry's unit was always so busy, anyway, that nobody really had time to do anything but take care of their patients. But this unit was special, and everyone had fun when they worked. The nurses loved their jobs, and Gerry knew she was loved by her nurses.

So, besides a lot of happy birthday wishes, it was a routine day in the Concentrated Care Unit. Then around two o'clock, Gerry got a call that there would be a short meeting with a few of the other head nurses on the second floor. Fine, Gerry thought. Then right after the meeting, she'd give report and leave.

The meeting was held in the conference room on the side of the building. It started late, but only lasted about a half hour. Afterwards, Gerry returned to her unit.

The first thing she saw were the balloons. There seemed to be hundreds of them, in all colors. Sayings were printed on them in magic marker like, "You Old Bat" and "Over the Hill." There were "Big 4-0" signs plastered all over the place, and multicolored streamers covered the nurses' station. There was a big sheet cake on the desk, and stacks of brightly wrapped presents piled up next to the cardiac monitors.

It was great! Gerry couldn't believe how quickly they had done all this! There were mobs of people there, all congratulating Gerry and hugging her. To top it off, Gerry was given a "crown" of a crazy hat complete with moose antlers, along with a decorated poesy to wear.

Everyone was loud and relaxed and eating cake. The nursing higher-ups never made rounds that late; after all, it was almost three o'clock. They were safe, Gerry thought.

It was at that exact moment when Gerry was dancing around in the middle of the nurses' station, flapping her "designer" poesy and wagging her antlers that the parade of administrators walked in. Led by the President/CEO of the hospital, the group of vice presidents, nursing executives, and entire Board of Trustees had chosen this hour to tour their hospital. There they were, right in the middle of all this craziness, staring at everyone and everything.

"Oh, my God. Oh, my God. Oh, my God," moaned Gerry, running into the medication room and slamming the door. Unfortunately, her best friend Annette was unable to follow. She had been secured into a chair with a tightly wrapped draw sheet, and her hands had been tied together behind her back with wrist restraints. Annette couldn't move. She couldn't speak either, since a piece of three inch adhesive tape had been placed tightly over her mouth. Annette just sat there with her eyes closed until she heard them leave.

Five minutes later, Gerry came out of the med room. "I know I'm fired," she said over and over again. "I know I'm fired." Just then, in walked Mrs. Lipton, the Vice President for Nursing. She came close to Gerry, who by this time was shaking.

"You're lucky these people have a sense of humor," she said quietly. "They thought this party was great." Mrs. Lipton then turned to leave. "By the way, Gerry," she said with a smile, "Happy Birthday!"

HARRY WOLF

Every spring and fall he was there.

The old timers had known him for years and expected him to be admitted to the Concentrated Care Unit at these times of the year. The new staff members had never met him, but once they did they never forgot him.

Harry Wolf had many medical problems, and his looks only made things worse. Harry had been burned many years before and his face was badly scarred. He had lost part of his scalp and so only tufts of hair covered his head.

Harry's admitting diagnoses were just about the same each time he was admitted. A non-compliant diabetic, Harry usually came in with sepsis, along with diabetic ketoacidosis. Sometimes he had pneumonia, and a few times the toes of his right foot had become gangrenous. He had an old colostomy and, since his skin care was so terrible, his bags never stayed on very well. Harry also suffered from chronic obstructive pulmonary disease, and required continuous low flow oxygen therapy.

Mr. Wolf was usually admitted late at night, and so his first nursing report was given by nights to the larger day staff. Due to his appearance, he was always given one of the few private rooms on the floor, even if it meant moving another patient. Harry's kardex was filled with orders and medications, and his care plan was long and involved. From the report, Harry did not sound like a great patient to take care of. He was nasty and withdrawn and spent most of his time in bed with the covers pulled up to cover his disfigured face. To top things off, Harry was always assigned to the newest nurse, one who hadn't met him before.

The day shift usually handled Harry Wolf the same way. After his new nurse met him, the laboratory was called to draw his blood. Respiratory therapy needed to give him a breathing treatment and the IV therapy team had to come to restart his infiltrated line. Radiology had to come up to do a portable chest x-ray and the dietary department had to bring him a late tray. And then, of course, the team of admitting residents needed to work Mr. Wolf up, so the first year resident had to come in to do his history and physical. Many people got to meet Harry Wolf, mostly in his darkened room with the shades drawn. One or two people were more than a bit startled.

Occasionally, Harry Wolf got a bit frisky. Someone would walk into the supply room or the nurses lounge and find the room pitch dark. When the light was turned on, there was Harry propped up in a wheelchair grinning a fiendish grin. He always seemed to enjoy shocking people.

Once a person met Harry, he or she would have a need to introduce him to someone else. A first year resident always called his second year for advice, and the IV nurse needed his or her partner to help find the vein. The x-ray tech needed assistance with technique, and the housekeeper needed her co-worker to bring in some more soap for the dispenser.

Yes, Harry Wolf was really something. One time the admitting registrar mistakenly spelled his name a different way. She took out the first "r" in Harry and put in an "i"" instead. And so Mr. Harry Wolf became Mr. Hairy Wolf, which described his rubber face completely.

That was back a few years ago during his spring admission, the first day of April. Or maybe it was in the fall, on the last day of October. And even today, when the tricksters play and the ghosts come out, Harry Wolf is admitted to the Concentrated Care Unit to meet the newest members of the hospital staff. Mr. Wolf truly is a legend.

THE GANG

He was hit on the head with some kind of metal pipe, maybe four or five times. His arm was in a sling and he was strapped to a backboard. Ronald, a member of a street gang, had been in a fight that day, and all this had happened in broad daylight. By the time the police arrived, nobody but Ronald was on the street. And, Ronald told them he had no idea who had hit him.

The initial x-rays showed a normal skull series and a fracture of his left shoulder. The CT department was not able to take him in right away, so Ronald was returned to the emergency department where he could be observed until it was time for him to be scanned. Since the cervical spine films were negative, Ronald now rested on a stretcher in one of the examining areas. He was drowsy, but responded easily.

Suddenly, after about fifteen minutes, Roanld sat up on the stretcher and looked around. Without a word, he jumped off the stretcher and ripped the sling off his broken shoulder and pulled out his IV. As a nurse and an orderly stood frozen, Ronald lowered his head and ran at top speed right into the wall. With his head taking the full force of the blow, he bashed into the wall as if he were trying to knock it down. The noise was terrifying.

As soon as Ronald hit the wall, his head snapped back and he fell to the floor. Then his body became rigid and he began to seize. At that point everyone came running. Ronald was rolled carefully on to the same backboard that he had been on earlier and his emergency care began again. After a while, the seizures stopped but Ronald no longer responded to any stimuli at all. He was brought back to x-ray and new pictures were taken of his cervical spine. Although it certainly appeared that Ronald could have broken his neck, the x-rays were negative. That was not the case, however, when the CT scan was done. There were multiple areas of hemorrhage throughout Ronald's brain.

By this time the emergency room was starting to fill with people, all who wanted to know what had happened to Ronald. One very upset young woman said she was his girlfriend, but the rest of the people identified themselves as friends. Most were very angry and a few acted outright threatening, yelling out loud about finding the "guy that did this." It got a little scary for the staff, who at that point had no idea what they should say or if, in fact, they should say anything at all about what had happened to Ronald while he was in the hospital.

Ronald, by now, was no longer breathing effectively on his own and he had been put on a respirator. It was time to send him up to the medical ICU, which now posed a huge problem with visitor control. It was obvious that most of the young people who had arrived in the emergency department were members of

Ronald's street gang, and they felt a very close bond with Ronald. They didn't want to be turned away. Gangs consider themselves family, and this was no exception.

By the time Ronald had been brought to the ICU, the staff up there had already formed a plan. They got Ronald settled and then the charge nurse, Roseanne, went out in the hall to talk to the crowd which had accumulated. A few security guards were standing silently along the wall, and they were obviously being ignored by the visitors. Roseanne told them how sick Ronald was and that while he was in the emergency room, he had been very restless and had banged his head, further increasing his head injury. She told them that the nurses knew just how important he was to them, but in a hospital there had to be rules in order for the patients to be cared for properly.

There needed to be one or two people who would act as spokesmen, and those would be the ones to whom all the information would be given. Right now, each of them would be allowed to see Ronald, but after that, visiting had to be limited. It was very obvious that this really was a family, every bit as close as if they were blood relatives. And somehow, Roseanne and the rest of the nurses knew that the gang was going to understand what had been said and to cooperate with the staff. And they did. They showed respect to the nurses and they followed the rules.

Maybe it was so easy because they saw the nursing staff in a position of authority and trusted them, just like they were used to doing with their own leaders. And maybe they somehow saw these nurses as "on their side." Whatever the reason, the only worry the staff had was if the person who had beat Ronald up would try to come back. There were city police and security guards stationed outside the unit around the clock, but there was never any trouble.

Ronald was pronounced brain dead, but since his vital signs were failing fast, no attempt was made to discontinue life support. Since he was an IV drug abuser, Ronald was not considered for organ donation. And, for legal reasons, the staff was told to call a code when Ronald's heart finally stopped.

When it was obvious that the end was near, extra police were brought in. They were never needed. And Ronald's friends, the big tough gang members, cried when the code was called, but they remained controlled and courteous.

The Medical Examiner's office took Ronald's body, but they were unable to say whether the cause of death was from the blows to the head from the metal pipe or from Roanld himself. Even though the person who hit him was found and charged with assault, he could not be charged with murder. Most likely though, later, the streets would have their own kinds of justice.

The Nursing staff, and much of the hospital in fact, learned from this. People are people, and if they are treated with respect and dignity, most will respond the same way. As different as we may be, we are very much the same.

LORETTA

She was used to being in control, after being a boss for so many years. Loretta had been the manager of a very busy department and was known for the tight ship she ran. What Loretta wanted her people to do, they did. Maybe not everyone loved her, but there was no question her place ran smoothly and her area was one of the most highly productive in the company. She had a lot of power.

Now the situation was totally different. After being diagnosed several years earlier with a progressively debilitating disease, Loretta was almost totally paralyzed. Whatever voluntary movements she had left were so limited that she could no longer do anything for herself. Loretta could move her left hand and foot only very slightly, and her breathing had become so weak that she needed help from a respirator.

But, Loretta remained one hundred per cent awake and alert and although she couldn't speak, she could still mouth words very clearly. Loretta never stopped "talking." She totally directed her care and told the staff exactly what she wanted and when and how she wanted it.

Now nobody could ever begin to imagine what it could be like for Loretta to be in a situation like that. It must have been horrible beyond anyone's imagination. Loretta's mind was literally locked up in a shell of a body. She was trapped, just as if she were locked away in a prison somewhere.

No nurse, after taking care of Loretta for a full shift wanted to take care of her again. Not only was she physically and emotionally draining, but Loretta came across as being selfish. Actually, she was a bitch. She was not a private duty patient and her nurses had a full district for which they were responsible. If they spent most of the shift in Loretta's room, they couldn't leave to go take care of their other patients.

Loretta didn't require any type of time consuming physical care. She needed to be bathed, positioned, tube fed, and suctioned. Add on some of the little extras, and there was still plenty of time for her nurse to leave and go tend to her other patients. But this never happened. After twenty minutes of propping her hand one way and positioning her ankle another way, and fluffing the pillow to a certain height, and folding the corner of the blanket at an exact angle, the nurse would turn and tell Loretta that she now had to leave to take care of her other patients. Loretta would then stare at the nurse and mouth the word, "bedpan," which meant another hour in that room of getting her just the way she wanted. And then she would ask for something else, just to keep the nurse there.

Now everyone knew that besides everything else, Loretta was probably scared to death. She was afraid to be alone, maybe fearing that she would pop off

69

the respirator and suffocate or something. All nurses know that demanding patients have reasons for their actions. Nurses know all the ways to deal with this and know all the behavior modification tricks. They tried coming in and checking on her every ten minutes. They attempted to anticipate her needs so she didn't have to ask for things. They gave her the little extras like putting makeup on her just the way she liked. In fact, makeup was even part of the written care plan.

But nothing worked. When the nurses told her that they had to leave to take care of another patient, Loretta stared them in the eyes and mouthed, "I don't care about any other patients. I just care about me, and I want you in this room."

So the real truth was that nobody could stand this sick lady. Maybe she just felt the world owed her something because she had developed this terrible disease. Maybe she was still in her anger stage and would eventually pass through it. Or maybe she was just a nasty self-centered person who only cared about herself. And, guess what? After taking care of her for weeks and weeks, nobody seemed to care about why she acted like she did. The only thing that concerned the nurses was that she was there. Day after day and evening after evening and night after night, she was always there.

Oh, forget about nursing challenges and all that fancy terminology garbage. The nurses began to take turns on a rotating basis just to be able to tolerate her. Nobody had easier days than anyone else. Even if a nurse spent extra time with her, it was not enough. Nothing was ever enough.

It was obvious that she wasn't going to get any better and go home, and she certainly didn't seem to be ready to die either. This was going to last and last. The head nurse went in and had a heart to heart talk with her. She told her kindly but very honestly just what was going on and how this was impacting on the unit and the staff. Loretta answered back just as honestly that she completely understood how very demanding she was and how she fully realized that she was taking nursing time from the other patients, but as she had said so often before, she really and truly didn't care. Or, as she so sweetly put it, "I really don't give a rat's ass about anybody else. That's not my problem. My problem is me."

So this went on and on and finally arrangements were made to send her home on the ventilator. This happened quite a few years ago, and patients with tracheostomies and ventilators just didn't leave the hospital back then. But Loretta was the first, at least at that hospital. When she left, she never even thanked anyone. Actually, she never even said good-bye. That day, the staff literally did a dance together right in the middle of the unit, celebrating their "freedom" and saying a little prayer for those home care nurses who would find out soon enough just what they had gotten themselves into.

For a month or so, life in the unit was good again. No matter how hard anybody had to work or how bad the shift was, there was no Loretta to make it worse.

Then one morning the floor got a call from the emergency room. Guess who was being admitted? It was Loretta, but she had suffered a stroke and was in a coma. Now this was different. In fact it was weird. Loretta was back, still on that respirator but now she was no longer in charge. The nurse had gotten back their control.

When she arrived on the unit and was put in bed it was a whole different ball game. Everybody came in to see her and even though she looked exactly the same, she still looked different. Although she certainly was alive, the life was out of her. The thing was, that nobody felt sorry for her at all. Why did they all feel that way, they wondered. Nurses, who are the most caring and most compassionate of the helping professions, always care. Don't they? Then how come, they asked, that no nurse, on any shift, could honestly say that there was even a fleeting feeling of "poor Loretta." To make it even more odd, nobody even felt a bit guilty for not having any sympathy. Some people, when they found out that she was unconscious, actually came out and said, "Good."

This really never had happened before. How did it get this far and this bad? Nobody cared. The only emotion anyone felt was satisfaction. Maybe Loretta had just gone too far. Maybe she had pushed people who do nothing but give of themselves too far across the line to be able to come back again. A least not yet. They say we should all be able to forgive, but maybe after being the way she was for so long that wasn't so easy to do. Loretta brushed on something in the nurses that is not usually touched and they just didn't want to remember any of those feelings any more.

A day later Loretta died. She was a DNR. The only thing felt then was relief that this finally was all over. For the nurses, more so than for Loretta.

WHY?

She had complained of a headache from the time she arrived at work that morning. She didn't feel well at all and she certainly didn't look right. Being four months pregnant, she was really afraid to take anything stronger than a Tylenol, and that just didn't seem to help.

Lucy worked in a very busy office with lots of little cubicles. She spent much of each day busy at her computer terminal, as did almost everyone else in the office. So when they first heard bumping, nobody really saw what was going on.

After about a minute of the strange sounds, the woman on the other side of Lucy's wall got up and walked around to see what the strange noise was. She found Lucy sprawled backward in her chair, having a grand mal seizure.

When the paramedics arrived, Lucy was still seizing. She had bitten her tongue and there was blood trickling from her mouth and down her chin. Lucy's eyes were rolled back in her head, and her color was bluish-white. The medics started an IV and got her out of there as fast as they possibly could.

The seizure was still in progress when Lucy arrived in the emergency department. No matter what drugs they gave her, it didn't break. Her teeth were clenched so tightly that her mouth could not be opened to release her tongue, which was still being bitten. Trying to pry her teeth apart would certainly break Lucy's jaw.

It was assumed that Lucy had suffered a massive intracerebral hemorrhage. After all, the headache and the seizing in a previously healthy young woman all painted that picture. Of course, the way to get such a diagnosis was a CT scan of the brain. Within five minutes they would have the answer, but Lucy had to stop seizing first. There was not way they could get her into the scanner and get any pictures until she was quiet.

It was one full hour later when Lucy finally stopped convulsing. By the time she had received more medication intravenously than it usually took to quiet four patients. Besides, Lucy was twenty-six years old and barely weighed a hundred pounds. Of course that little baby had also received these huge quantities of drugs, but right now the race was to save the mother.

When Lucy was finally lifted from the stretcher to the CT table, she left behind sheets soaked with blood. They had found, when they finally opened her mouth, that her tongue had been bitten almost in two. There had been no time to worry about the tongue, since by this time Lucy appeared almost dead. She was no longer breathing and was being ventilated by a respirator through a tube down her nose into her trachea. The left pupil was twice the size of the right one, and neither reacted to light. Lucy's heart rhythm was very irregular with lots of dangerous beats.

The CT scanning room was crowded with people watching the pictures come across the screen, all expecting to see the characteristic white blotches in the brain which represent patches of blood. But the scan was normal. Nothing. No bleeding. No swelling. Nothing but normal brain tissue.

The nurses pulled Lucy off the scanning table and back onto the stretcher, which had now been covered with clean white sheets. They ran with her from the CT department up towards the medical ICU. and by the time they reached the elevator the new clean sheets were once again drenched with blood. It really was a blessing that her husband and parents, who were still in the emergency department, weren't there to see this.

Almost immediately after Lucy was placed in the ICU bed, her heart began to fibrillate and then, even before it could be shocked, the heart came to a standstill. Besides the code team, a page went out for any cardiologist in the house, since now the thought was that Lucy may have suffered a massive heart attack. There must have been three times the normal number of people at that code. Three cardiologists had responded along with a pulmonologist and an anesthesiologist. Everyone was working to save this girl. In a last ditch effort to reverse what could have been an overwhelming flood of blood clots to the lung, they gave her drugs to try to dissolve them.

They worked for one hour. Lucy's parents did not want to come into the unit, but the nurse brought her husband in to see the frantic effort to save Lucy's life four times. He just had to see what was happening and each time he was brought in by two nurses, each holding on to him. One of the ICU nurses called up to obstetrics to tell them that the code and all the STAT pages was for a young pregnant girl, but when the OB staff found out that the fetus was only four months old, they knew there was nothing to be done.

Finally it was all over. Everybody was sobbing with the family. Lucy's mother fainted. It was just about the worst code most of the seasoned ICU nurses had ever seen.

The medical examiner released Lucy's body. In big cities, they just don't have time to autopsy every case like this. The coroner only takes violent or really suspicious deaths. Here the cause of death was, most probably, a massive heart attack or pulmonary emboli. But why did this happen to a twenty-six year old? Nobody knew.

The family refused an autopsy, and it was their right to do so. The nurses, crying openly, gave Lucy's body a bath and washed her hair. She had a tiny little belly, just staring to show. When the family came in to say good-bye for the last time, Lucy's hair was blond and clean again. The hardest part was when they took her wedding and engagement rings off her hand and gave them to the young husband.

For the rest of that week, everyone thought of Lucy. That night her girlfriends probably called her to talk. What do you say when someone asks to speak to Lucy? Do you say that she's dead? It was so fast, so sudden. What do you tell people?

Nobody knows why tragedies like this happen. And, nothing like these types of tragedies bring nurses closer to each other and to their own friends and families. As somebody once said, in a blink of an eye the world stops and when it starts again, everything is different. And nobody on earth knows why.

"LUKE THE PUKE"

He was an all around great guy. The best. He was everyone's favorite medical resident and cardiology fellow. Smart. Caring. Sensitive. Loving. And funny. Always funny. "Remember to write your pulmonary artery pressures on scraps of paper towels and then lose the towel so you don't have the numbers to chart," he'd advise the scared new ICU nurses. Then he'd laugh when they just nodded seriously at him. You just couldn't say enough about Dr. Jim. The nurses loved him and the attending physicians respected him. He was just bound to do well in life.

And he did. He started his practice in cardiology and before long it was booming. The other doctors referred their patients to him and the nurses raved about him to anyone who asked for a cardiologist. Dr. Jim married his college sweetheart, and by the time he finished his fellowship, they had four beautiful little children. He was so proud of his family, and he brought the kids in often on weekends when he made rounds. They all looked like him and it was obvious how much they adored him. Life was good.

Then one day Dr. Jim got a new machine in his office. A new toy, he called it. Instead of sending his patients' blood out to private labs, they could run their own blood counts. It would be easier for the patients that way, he felt. Answer would come back immediately and the patients could be treated better and faster.

The office staff tried it first. They drew blood on each other and then used the new toy to see the results. Of course everyone was normal. "Don't tell me you're tired because you're anemic," joked Dr. Jim. "Everyone here is perfect."

But, when Dr. Jim put his own blood in the new toy, something seemed strange. His white blood count was very high. "That's funny," thought Dr. Jim. "I'm not sick or anything. I feel fine." So he waited until the next day and repeated the blood work. The white count was even higher. Now Dr. Jim got scared.

He went to his friend, Cathy Henderson, who was a hematologist. They had been medical residents together and had remained close. He told Cathy that he was really scared and was afraid that he had something horrible. Cathy repeated the blood count in her office and the number was still the same. It was time for a bone marrow aspiration to find out what was going on. When Cathy came to Dr. Jim to tell him the results, she didn't even have to say a word. They both knew. She hugged him and they cried together. Leukemia.

Right then and there, Dr. Jim's life began to change. His heaven on earth broke to little pieces there in that office and his two year fight to live began.

75

Unlike children, who now have great chances of cure, adult leukemia is not in the same league. At least not the type of leukemia that Dr. Jim had.

All through his chemotherapy, Dr. Jim continued to work. Sick as a dog and with his shiny black hair getting thinner and duller, he saw patients in the office and made rounds in the hospital. The CCU nurses remember Dr. Jim continuing to make jokes with them and worry about the patients. Life had to go on, he said.

Dr. Jim's remission lasted less than eight months. He knew he had relapsed before he saw the lab work. He could just tell, he said. He felt different, and it wasn't the chemo this time that was making him sick. It was the disease. It was "Luke the Puke," as he called it. Dr. Jim's only chance to live was a bone marrow transplant.

All four of his brothers were tested and none of them was a match. The family was devastated. Other relatives were tested and nobody came close. Dr. Jim was on staff at four different hospitals and was loved by everyone who knew him, so when the search for a bone marrow donor was made public, there was such an overwhelming response that it was almost unbelievable. The line to get into the building where the drive was held wrapped around the block. Literally thousands of people were tested. Surely one of them would be able to help, even if it wasn't a perfect match. Right?

But this was not the way it turned out. Nobody came near. Dr. Jim knew there was nothing left for him, but he continued to take care of his patients. They knew he was sick. It was obvious. Everyone knew he was sick. His walk was slower and he ached all over from the drugs he took every day. But Dr. Jim often said that if he ever stopped doing what he loved, that would mean he had given in to his disease, and he was not ready to give in yet.

One of the ICU nurses had a niece who had leukemia and Dr. Jim continued to ask about her all the time. JoAnn had been in remission for two years and his face always lit up when he heard how well she was doing. "She'll beat "Luke the Puke," he smiled. That was the last thing she remembered Dr. Jim saying, because that night he began to vomit blood and was admitted to the ICU.

At the end of the week, Dr. Jim surrendered to his disease. He had received countless units of blood and platelets and plasma, and finally he said that was enough. Dr. Jim told his doctors that he didn't want to use any more of the valuable blood products which other cancer patients needed. As he put it, "it only comes out as fast as you put it in, and it's being wasted on me. I just want to go home. I give up."

That same day Dr. Jim went home. Two of the nurses and two of the doctors who were his friends and colleagues were with him when he died. He was at home in his own bed surrounded by his family. "Luke the Puke" had won.

LAVERNE AND SHIRLEY

They were best friends and had been so since high school. After graduating from nursing school together, they decided to work at the same hospital on the same evening shift. Each was a bridesmaid at the other's wedding, and their husbands and kids had become friends.

They had all of the same tastes and likes, and their very favorite television show was "Laverne and Shirley." In fact, they had a standing request to be off on Tuesdays so that they could be home to watch their show. Everyone kidded them and soon they became know as Laverne and Shirley.

One day Shirley told Laverne that for the past week she had been having lots of abdominal cramps with some bloody diarrhea. But she wasn't worried, she said. After all, she was only thirty-two years old so it really couldn't be anything terrible. Not cancer or anything like that. Thirty-two year olds don't get colon cancer, she said. It most likely was an onset of some kind of inflammatory bowel disorder or an attack of colitis which was sure to subside. If it didn't go away or if it got worse, she would see a doctor. But what could he tell her that she didn't know already, anyway? She'd go on a bland diet and wait it out. She knew all these doctors and she would never let them stick anything up her behind, she said. She knew exactly what they would find. After all, she was an experienced nurse and could figure out what was wrong with her.

Shirley made Laverne promise to keep her mouth shut and Laverne agreed to do so, as long as Shirley would let her know if she didn't get better. That was the deal these best friends made. By the second week, she was fine again. At least that's what Shirley told Laverne.

One evening Laverne was at work when she got a call that Shirley was out on the emergency ramp in the car with her husband. Shirley was doubled over in pain and couldn't stand up. The emergency room staff ran out and bundled Shirley onto a stretcher and wheeled her into the department.

Shirley was, by this time, in shock with a perforated bowel. The emergency surgery showed that Shirley's large intestine had been perforated by a rapidly growing and invasive cancerous tumor which had eaten its way through the bowel wall. The surrounding lymph nodes were involved and the cancer had spread into the pelvis. A colostomy was done but the tumor was not able to be resected.

Three months and many tears later, Shirley came back to work. After all, she loved nursing and wanted to be doing what made her happy. But this didn't last very long. Ten days after her return to work, Shirley was readmitted to the hospital. She was in awful pain and her abdomen was grossly distended with fluid. Shirley had begun to die.

The chemotherapy had not touched the cancer. It was, in fact, growing like crazy. Now Shirley was put on a morphine drip in an attempt to make her more comfortable. Every evening when Laverne's shift was over she came and sat with Shirley, just holding her hand and listening to her talk.

One evening when Shirley's breathing had become labored, Laverne came in and said, "Shirley, I've come to cry with you now." They both cried together for a long time and then Shirley told Laverne about her terrible fear. She said she had a recurring dream that after she died she would still be able to hear things, and she was afraid that after she was buried she would hear the dirt being shoveled onto the top of her coffin. She would go crazy, she said. She was more afraid of that than anything else.

Laverne told her that she absolutely knew that Shirley would not be able to hear anything after she died. She told Shirley to believe her -- that she had always told her the truth and she would never lie to her now. Somehow, that made Shirley feel safer and she was able to sleep. When the phone rang early that next morning, Laverne knew what had happened. Shirley had died a few hours earlier while she slept.

There was an honor guard of nurses at Shirley's funeral. They came in their white uniforms and Shirley's body was carried out through the double line of nurses down the steps of the funeral home and into the hearse. There was a letter in the coffin to Shirley from Laverne, a letter which reminded Shirley that if she could hear anything at all, it was only the ripples of Laverne's love. And the letter was signed with a big "L," just like the one Laverne wore on her sweaters on the T.V. show.

Now, eighteen years later, Laverne often thinks of her friend Shirley when people speak of the old television shows. And when "Laverne and Shirley" is mentioned, Laverne looks up toward the sky and shares a secret smile with her forever best friend.

GOOD-BYE BEN

For most of his twenty-six years, Ben had suffered with some type of serious medical problem. Diagnosed as a diabetic when he was only five years old, Ben soon began to suffer from complications of the disease.

By the time he was a teenager, Ben already had high blood pressure and at the age of twenty the circulation to his legs and feet had become compromised. A few years, later Ben had developed problems with his vision and his kidneys had begun to fail.

Ben was a clinic patient and followed all the medical advice to the letter. The nursing staff in the different clinics loved Ben. He was a gentleman and a little boy all at the same time. He wanted so much to live a normal healthy life and he tried so hard. But no matter what he did or the doctors and nurses did, Ben's condition continued to worsen. His body seemed about thirty years older than it really was.

Ben tolerated just about everything that happened to him, but his one fear was that his kidneys would shut down enough that he would have to go on dialysis. For whatever reason, this meant the end of the line for Ben. He always said that if this day came, he would just give up.

Everyone knew how Ben felt about dialysis. Everything else was tried first, but finally there was no other way. Without dialysis to help his body get rid of its toxins, there would be much more damage done.

Nobody wants to become dependent on an artificial kidney. To be committed to a machine for four hours per day three times per week means that the person's life now revolves around dialysis. This is extremely hard on anyone.

But with Ben, it meant more. The hemodialysis represented failure on his part ... failure to have control over the disease. So when Ben was about to begin his treatments, the entire staff became very worried about him. Once he was started and put on a schedule, Ben was to begin counseling to help him cope.

But the clinic staff admitted Ben to the hospital because they became so worried about him. He was more than sad; he was actually despondent. Ben had a dual lumen dialysis catheter placed and was scheduled for his first treatment that next morning. It was going to be a long night for Ben.

The last time the night nurse checked on Ben he was asleep. Then the night shift ended and the day shift arrived for report. There was a long delay during report when nobody made rounds, which is common practice in all hospitals.

Report ended and the day nurse started to make her first rounds. Ben wasn't in his bed and she assumed he was in the bathroom. The nurse then left his room and continued on down the hall.

About fifteen minutes later the staff heard the cleaning lady screaming. It was coming from Ben's bathroom. They ran down the hall towards the door which was now open. Blood was everywhere. The rubber tip of the dialysis catheter had been pulled off, and since it was positioned in a major blood vessel, it hadn't taken very long for him to loose much of his blood supply right through the open port.

Ben was lying on the floor in the bathroom. He was dead. There was a note in the sink, written in magic marker on a paper towel, which simply said,

"I'M SORRY."

Well, of course there was an investigation and of course everyone was questioned. Patients just don't commit suicide in hospitals. Certainly there was guilt and certainly there was all the "maybe we could have's" and "maybe we should have's." In the end it was just called a tragedy that couldn't have been prevented. And it really couldn't.

The clinic nurses sent a big floral wreath to Ben's wake. Several of them attended the funeral to say good-bye and all of them whispered the same thing to Ben's body.

"I'M SORRY TOO."

TOGETHER

They had made a pact, back then. He was going to die in their bed, and she would be with him. When the time was right, one or both of them would know. And, she would get into bed with him and she would hold him while he died.

Danny was only thirty years old. Diagnosed with Hodgkin's Disease, he was given a pretty good chance to be cured at the beginning. Even then, when cancer treatments certainly were not as sophisticated as they are now, Hodgkin's Disease was considered one of the "good ones." The treatment might be tough, but he should live. They had great hopes.

Danny was treated at one of the biggest and best medical centers in New York City, if not the world. He got the same therapies that all the other people with the same diagnosis received. Their cancers shrunk and they went right into remission. Most of them stayed that way. Danny's disease didn't budge. His cancer did not seem to be affected at all. The disease continued to spread and soon went from a stage one to a stage four. Soon most of the nodes in his chest and abdomen were involved.

The oncologists fought this with all the ammunition they had, but for some unexplainable reason, Danny's disease only progressed. There was nothing else. So Danny and his wife Sarah, made their pact. They had been "in love" since kindergarten and even back then, they knew they were going to get married and spend their lives together. They lived in a small suburb of New York City.

Danny and Sarah had gotten married at the age of twenty-two and had two beautiful little girls. They had bought a little house in the same town in which they had grown up, and their children now attended their same elementary school. In fact, the kids had the same teachers that had been there for Danny and Sarah. It was just like in a story book.

As always, Danny and Sarah faced life together. There was no such thing as pretending for each other or trying to be brave. As they had always done, they were in this as one, and not two separate people. If Danny had to die, they would be together for that also.

This was before the time of Hospice, so they were on their own. But that was okay; that was the way they wanted it. They just needed each other to do this. Danny's mother had remained very close all through this ordeal, and she, like all the rest of their family, supported their decision.

Well, finally, after almost two years, it seemed as if the time was here. One evening Danny began to die. He was at home, just like they planned. Sarah was there and so was Danny's mother. Danny was in his bed, but his dying was not like they thought it would be. They both believed that Danny would simply fall into a deep sleep and not wake up, and that would be the end. But nobody had prepared them for what else could happen.

Instead of the peaceful sleep that they both expected, Danny's breathing became very labored. His lungs filled with fluid and he felt as if he were drowning. Danny became restless and confused and he started to thrash around trying to get out of bed. His color was bluish. Sarah and Danny's mother got very scared. They didn't know what to do. So they called the police.

Well, you can figure out what happened after that. The police called an ambulance and Danny was rushed to the emergency department of the local hospital. After just a short time in the emergency room, Danny had a bunch of needles and tubes in him. He had received a ton of medications, and he was on a respirator. But, once again, he was awake and now he found himself in the exact condition he feared so much. He didn't want to die in a hospital. He wanted to die at home, in bed with Sarah. Of course, Sarah now felt as if she had betrayed Danny, and that all of this was her fault.

Danny was brought up to the ICU. Sarah followed him into the room and found him lying in his own diarrhea. Although Danny couldn't speak, tears of frustration and disgust ran down his face. How could all of this have happened?

The nurses decided that this was not going to be the way Danny died. He was going to die at home, in his own bed, with Sarah at his side, just the way they had wanted it. Right then and there the planning and the conferences began. Given the right medications and IV fluids, Danny was thankfully able to be weaned off the respirator. Once that was done, it was time to get him home.

This time, Danny was sent home on lots of sedation and pain medication, and most of all support. Twice a day a phone call was made to Sarah to answer questions and just to listen. Sarah knew where to call when she needed to ask something or just to hear a familiar voice. What Hospice nurses do every day today, the ICU nurses did back then. And it worked.

When Danny's real time came to die, he just got sleepier and sleepier. When his breathing became irregular and very slow, Sarah just knew. She got into bed with Danny and held him in her arms and told him how much she loved him, and how she would never ever leave him. Sarah just held on to Danny, even after she felt his guardian angel take him and carry him up to heaven. This was the way it was meant to be.

FRIENDS 4-EVER

They met during Rosie's twenty-fifth hospitalization, when she was getting ready for her thirteenth operation. When she had her baseball cap on, the only thing that made Rosie seem any different from any other sixteen year old kid was the fact that she had no eyelashes or eyebrows.

This was Joan's third time in the hospital since she had begun her chemotherapy, and each admission was because she started to run fevers due to her low white blood count. Joan really didn't feel very sick but she had to stay in the hospital for intravenous antibiotics. That was the way they did things when kids on chemo got fevers. Routine.

Joan had acute lymphoblastic leukemia, a disease that while always fatal not so long ago, now has a cure rate of over 70 percent. Rosie had Wilm's Tumor, a type of kidney cancer that little kids get. Wilm's is also highly curable today, but this wasn't the case for Rosie. Rosie had been diagnosed fifteen years ago when she was only one year old, and despite all the chemo and surgeries she had endured, the cancer kept coming back. In fact she now was going to have part of her remaining lung removed to try to cut out more of that recurring cancer.

Joan was fifteen when she met Rosie, and before that first day ended they knew everything there was to know about each other. In fact, fate had made them roommates and they stayed up that whole preop night talking. They talked not about illness, but about what normal teenage girls think about. Boys. School. Boys. Clothes. Boys.

Rosie's body was crisscrossed with surgical scars, and catheters from her implanted chemotherapy port stuck out of her chest. But, since Rosie dressed in sweat pants and sweatshirts all the time, nobody could see any of this. She was just Rosie.

Joan waited that next day for the surgery to be over and, as Rosie told her it would happen, she waited to hear the doctors and nurses come in and tell her that now Rosie's cancer was all gone and she was cured. But Rosie didn't come back to her room after surgery, since she had gone to the intensive care unit. That was expected, the nurses told Joan. After all, she had undergone major chest surgery. Joan was watching television in her room when Rosie's mother came in to talk to Joan's mother.

Joan came right out and asked Rosie's mom if Rosie was now cured of cancer. No, she was told. Rosie knew she wasn't going to be cured. Ever. She knew this surgery was just going to give her a little more time, but she knew she was going to die. Probably within just a few months. Didn't Rosie tell Joan this?

Joan got out of her bed and walked down the hall into the playroom. She looked around and studied the unit. It looked like a place for kids, that's all. There were toys and games for the little ones and computers and V.C.R.'s for the older kids. Except for the fact that lots of the kids were bald and had IV's running, nobody seemed to be very sick. There was lots of noise and laughter. There were play ladies and volunteers and families everywhere. The "candy man" was rolling his cart up and down the hall, giving out ice pops and lolly pops and popcorn to anyone who wanted something. This was not a place for dying, but a place where a lot of living was going on.

Joan had never really thought about dying. There never was any question in her mind that she would be fine after her two and a half years of chemotherapy ended. Chemotherapy. The word itself meant treatment with medicine. Didn't medicine make you better? That's what she always thought happened. So why would Rosie, who was just like her, go through all those years of operations and treatment if it wasn't going to work anyway?

She had a really hard time sleeping that night. Besides the fact that her temperature was up and she felt achy all over, she had too much on her mind. Joan felt as if she had known Rosie her whole life. She was like one of her best friends, and she was sure if they had met at another time and another place, they would have been very close. They were so much alike. So, how could Rosie really be dying? And, why hadn't she said anything about it? Even at fifteen, Joan knew the answer to that one. Rosie obviously didn't want to deal with it.

The next day, Rosie was back from intensive care, and she began to feel better fast. Within two days, all her tubes were out and she was again walking around and in good spirits. That afternoon, one of the activities of the floor was decorating baseball caps. Rosie and Joan made the hats say:

"Rose and Joan -- Best Friends 4-Ever"

Then each gave each other the hat she had made. Joan never approached Rosie about her future. They talked about going to each other's high school graduation and being a bridesmaid in each other's wedding. And, they planned to go to nursing school together. Each wanted to be a pediatric hematology-oncology nurse and show other kids with cancer that they can get through their treatment. The next day Joan was discharged, and Rosie was due to go home the day afterward. They exchanged addresses and promised they would write to each other.

Joan and Rosie met once more by chance in the clinic, where each had gone for follow-up appointments. Rosie looked thinner and had a terrible cough. She told Joan she had been fighting a lot with her mother because "my mother has a hard time dealing with the fact that my disease is considered fatal." Then Rosie immediately changed the subject to going to nursing school and Joan never tried to change it back.

About six weeks later, Rosie's mother called Joan's house to say that Rosie had died. Joan couldn't even go to the funeral because she was back in the hospital again with more fevers. But, Joan said good-bye to Rosie, alone one night in the darkened playroom at the big table where they had sat making their "Friends-4 -Ever" hats. She knew Rosie was listening.

That was six years ago, Joan is now a senior in nursing school, and still plans on being a pediatric hematology-oncology nurse. She is now considered a long term survivor of leukemia and is very active in the Leukemia Society. When Joan graduated from high school, she dedicated her yearbook memories to her friend Rosie, who she just knew was up there in heaven organizing the best parties and activities for all other angels. And no matter what the future brings, Joan and Rosie will be friends 4-ever.

THOMAS AND JULIA

He really needed new glasses, he told Julia. His eyesight was getting worse and worse. Things were pretty blurry, actually. It had been several years since he'd last had his eyes examined and he guessed it was time for a checkup.

Thomas made the appointment with his eye doctor for the next week. There was no rush, actually. He'd been having problems for quite a while now, and a few weeks more wouldn't make any difference.

Julia and Thomas had been married for just five years. They say love is lovelier the second time around, and for them this was absolutely true. Both had been married before, and now they had a one year old toddler. A big beautiful boy, Kevin, was the pride of both of them. He looked exactly like Thomas. They were the perfect all American family.

Thomas, a high school music teacher, went to see the eye doctor, expecting to hear that he needed a new prescription for glasses. But, that wasn't what the doctor told him. It seemed that the eye exam showed an increase in pressure in Thomas' head. Something was wrong and Thomas needed to see a neurologist right away.

Julia had been a critical care nurse for years and knew almost all the doctors on staff at her hospital. That same afternoon, Julia and Thomas got an appointment and were seen by the neurologist. There was indeed a problem. They had to find out what was going on, and they needed to do so quickly.

The next morning, Thomas went for testing. Magnetic resonance imaging showed a tumor, and a fairly large one at that. The sophisticated MRI pointed to a pituitary adenoma, a type of tumor which is almost always benign, yet needed to be treated immediately. Like any type of brain tumor, it could not be left to grow. The skull leaves no room for anything to expand, and allowing it to do so could only cause damage to the brain. In Thomas' case, the vision center was already being affected.

Thomas and Julia's picture perfect world started to turn upside down. He needed to have surgery as soon as possible, and would be a patient in Julia's own surgical intensive care unit. This type of tumor grows in the base of the brain, and surgery is usually long and tedious.

Julia had been part of this unit for many years, and the nursing staff was family to her. Julia knew that Thomas was not only going to get the best care, but also a lot of love. She had the doctors and nurses that she knew and trusted, along with the comfort of her home away from home. And, Thomas trusted Julia and her decisions completely.

This was a very hard time for Julia. They say ignorance is bliss, and now more than ever this rang true. It is very difficult to be a wife and a nurse at the same time, and extremely hard to separate the two. Julia had been a nurse too long. She knew what should happen and what could happen. Trying to be strong for Thomas, Julia needed to be taken care of herself. Her husband had a brain tumor. She needed to cry and be scared, not to be the strong reassuring nurse to all of Thomas' friends and family. Julia needed her own kind of care.

The day of the surgery came, and as soon as Thomas left for the operating room, Julia began to cry. She cried for a while, and then she sat and waited. But, instead of sitting in the waiting room like other visitors, she stayed in the surgical ICU with her nursing family. They took care of her, just as if she were one of their patients. So when, twelve hours after the surgery ended, Julia was told that Thomas needed to return to the operating room again because his brain had swelled, Julia was unable to handle that also.

Finally, it was over. Most of the tumor, but not all, had been removed. Time would tell if his eyesight, which now was minimal, would ever return. It was a waiting game. After a stay in the ICU, Thomas was transferred to a regular room and then, after just a few days, he was discharged home. Julia took some time off to be with Thomas. He couldn't see well enough to be able to take care of the baby, and after all, he still needed some taking care of himself.

The doctors wanted to wait until most of the swelling in the brain had gone down in order to decide if radiation therapy would help Thomas. Thomas, always the cheerful one, told Julia that his eyesight was improving. But Julia knew better. She could see how he faked things, how he made believe he was reading or watching television. But, she knew her husband too well.

Thomas started on a course of radiation therapy. Every day for six weeks, Thomas came to the hospital for his treatments, and every day they waited for his vision to improve. The radiologists told Thomas that radiation usually stops the growth of the tumor forever, and hopefully would shrink whatever was left of it, enough for his vision to improve. Julia and Thomas knew that any results would happen very slowly and they just had to take one day at a time.

The follow-up MRI showed a dramatic decrease in the size of the remaining tumor, which was wonderful news. Over the next few months, Thomas' vision improved slightly in one eye and he is now able to read and once again see his sheet music. Thomas is still out on medical disability but hopes to be able to return to his teaching job next year. His students and the other teachers miss him a lot.

Life goes on, although it may be different. Julia and Thomas realize just how precious their time together is. And, Julia's medical and nursing colleagues knew that more was involved in the healing process than just Thomas' physical needs. Julia, who was so used to being the care giver, needed to be taken care of also. It was a package deal.

QUEEN BESSIE

"Bessie's back."

Those two words were repeated over and over again during those years when Bessie Rivers was a patient in their hospital. Bessie was a regular, and was one of the first respirator dependent patients they ever sent home. In fact, they remember how they first weaned Bessie from the big ventilator and tried her on what they referred to as the "bedside baby." Bessie loved the fuss, and never felt afraid of the change. She trusted the staff completely and knew they'd never leave her on anything unreliable.

Bessie became a fixture in the unit. Really a medical patient, Bessie routinely was admitted to the surgical side. When the new building had gone up a few years ago, the staff of the old floors was redistributed and most of those who had been Bessie's nurses had gone to the surgical unit. Everyone knew Bessie belonged to them, and there was no question as to where to admit her.

Having to go back to the hospital never bothered Bessie. In fact she spent much more time in the hospital than at home. She referred to her times of discharge as "road trips," knowing full well that she would be back very soon.

Bessie had long-standing emphysema, as well as severe osteoporosis. She probably weighed about eighty pounds. With her long gray hair hanging down over her permanent tracheostomy, Bessie sat propped up in bed with the pillows arranged just as she liked them. Bessie suctioned herself and fed herself her meals. She kept her bedpan next to the bed and got herself on and off as she needed it. When it needed emptying, Bessie called someone, but otherwise she did her own care. All she needed was someone to fill her wash basin and set her up.

Her hospitalizations were usually due to pneumonia which, during the last two years of her life, occurred more and more frequently. There was a DNR order on her chart, but even without it nobody would ever dream of coding Bessie. Her ribs would crunch to dust as soon as anyone tried CPR. She was that fragile.

Bessie knew everything about "her nurses" and their lives. Her husband and son regularly brought birthday presents and cards for them, and she laughed at the goings on of their children. In fact, she had pictures of them up on her bulletin board. She was family. One of the doctors remembered that when he was a little boy he used to play with Bessie's son. He had memories of her walking them to school with her long brown hair blowing in the breeze and a Pall Mall cigarette dangling from her mouth.

Nurses took turns checking on Bessie when she was home, but there never was any problem. She ran her house from her "bedside baby" ventilator. She was the queen. In fact, that was what the nurses called her. Queen Bessie. They called her that to her face, and she loved it. In the hospital, she was completely in charge of her care, and that was fine with everyone. Nobody meddled with Queen Bessie. She was the boss.

Well, one night when they heard the familiar, "Bessie's back," things were different. This time Bessie had had a stroke and she was dying. She was in a coma. Bessie came up to "her unit" and "her nurses" arranged Bessie's room just the way she always liked it. Even though they knew she would never go home again, they kept Bessie on her "bedside baby" ventilator, instead of putting her back on one of the regular big ones.

In the two days before Bessie died, her nurses talked to her constantly, telling her all the latest details of their lives. It had always seemed that Bessie was immortal, that nothing could ever happen to her. Bessie had lived so many years at the same level and she had really become a big part of them. They were going to miss her, and they told her that. Even though Bessie was unconscious, they all were sure she could hear what they were saying.

So Bessie passed away, right there in her other home with "her nurses" all around her. It really wasn't sad. Even in death she looked like a queen, lying in her bed surrounded by everything she loved. Queen Bessie would never be forgotten in that unit. She was one special lady.

SECTION FOUR

OUT OF THE ORDINARY

JUST ANOTHER NIGHT SHIFT

It was late in the evening when Mrs. Emerson died. Her son had left the hospital about an hour earlier, after having spent most of the day with his mother. Receiving the phone call, Mr. Emerson returned to the room. He spent about ten minutes with his mother's body, talking to her quietly and saying good-bye.

Toni and Marion, two of the nurses on duty that night, were standing in the hall waiting for Mr. Emerson. It was then that the bat flew out of the open ceiling tile. It soared over their heads and into the room, landing on the headboard of the dead woman's bed. Mr. Emerson had just turned away to leave when he heard the two nurses scream and realized what happened.

It was a scene from "Dracula" -- a bat hovering over a dead body. The only difference was that this was a brightly lit modern nursing unit. The two nurses instantly took off and raced down the hall, leaving Mr. Emerson, his dead mother, and the bat.

Suddenly the bat left the headboard and flew back out into the hall. Mr. Emerson, without a second's hesitation, grabbed a sheet off the linen cart, swung it around, and whipped that bat down right out of the air. It lay twitching on the ground and then was still.

Toni and Marion, from the safety of the medication room, saw what had happened. Mr. Emerson, his head down, walked slowly down the hall past the nurses' station. Goodnight," he said sadly, as if absolutely nothing had happened. "Thank you all for taking such good care of my mother."

THE WORM

They called him Jake. He was a young man, not more than twenty-five or so. Jake had arrived in the United States only two weeks ago and he had planned to live with his brother and his family until could get settled on his own. Jake came from a very small and very poor country where times were hard.

A week after his arrival, Jake had gotten sick and had steadily become worse. By the time he was admitted to the hospital, he was ill enough to need the intensive care unit. After much testing, Jake was diagnosed with a liver abscess.

One afternoon, Jake felt worse. He was nauseated and told his brother he was going to vomit. Jake's brother went out to get Katie, who was his nurse. Katie stood at Jake's bedside with an emesis basin, holding it while Jake retched. Nothing but clear mucus came up.

Katie describes what happened next as the most horrible experience of her life. She was about to put the emesis basin down when suddenly Jake started to gag. A long brown worm came up into Jake's mouth and dropped out into the emesis basin. The worm moved ever so slightly, but it definitely moved. It was about six inches long and it was alive.

Well, forget about professionalism. Forget about reassurance and compassion. Katie lost it. She let out a scream which could be heard all over the unit. She whirled around with the basin in her hand and tossed it across the room towards the little sink in the corner. Somehow both the worm and the basin landed in the sink, and as Katie put it later, it sure was lucky that she didn't toss it right into the patient's face since that's what almost happened. Katie ran out of the room. When the other nurses reached Katie, she was leaning on the wall outside in the hall, pale and drenched with sweat. She kept repeating, "A worm. A worm. He threw up a worm."

Poor Jake. And poor Jake's brother. Jake's brother looked like he himself was going to faint and Jake just lay there with his eyes closed. Maybe he was too sick to know what happened or even to care.

Well, the worm was sent to pathology as per policy when anything is removed from the body. Of course, nobody would touch the worm to put it in the specimen jar but one brave person covered it with something so it couldn't get out of the sink or crawl down the drain hole. Who picked it up out of the sink and put it in a specimen jar? It was the gastroenterologist himself, who didn't seem at all horrified. In fact, he casually announced that these worms are called "ascariasis," and are not uncommon in underdeveloped countries where people eat spoiled and undercooked food. This worm, and others like it, he told the staff, had probably taken up residence in this patient's duodenum or jejunum. Delightful. Wonderful. Perfect.

No more little visitors made their appearance while Jake was in the ICU. This was especially reassuring since the nursing staff learned that the larva of these worms could migrate through the wall of the small intestine and be carried by the lymphatics and bloodstream to the lungs. What if one good cough brought forth another little pet?

Jake was treated with oral medications to kill the worms, and that was that. His liver abscess, which was now thought to have been caused by worms or larva in the billiary ducts, slowly resolved with treatment. Jake was soon out of intensive care and discharged home with his brother. If any worms remained in Jake's body, their remains most likely spent the next month or so circulating in the sewer system of the state of New Jersey.

UNDER THE DRESSING

Mr. Callahan was a whiner. In fact, that's exactly what the nurses named him. They called him Mr. Whiner. Oh, not to his face of course. But, when he rang that bell, they would say, "Oh, look. It's Mr. Whiner calling again." When they left his room after answering his light, they would sigh and ask, "Guess what Mr. Whiner wanted this time?"

Mr. Callahan complained about everything, and he did so in a very annoying sing-song voice. "Why do I have to sit up in that chair again?" he would ask. Or, he would ask questions that just didn't have any real answers, like "Why are hospitals always so cold?" And he moaned out loud all the time. When he was asked why he was moaning, he would answer in his sniveling little voice, "I'm not moaning. I'm just so uncomfortable." He sounded just like that nerd, Steve Urkel on the television show, "Family Matters."

Nobody could pass Mr. Callahan's room without hearing his annoying little groaning voice calling out to them for something stupid, like "Why are these sheets so rough on my skin?" He was just a pain in the neck.

Mr. Callahan had undergone surgery for a colon resection three days earlier and, aside from all the whining, he was doing very well. The staff on all three shifts couldn't wait till he recovered and went home.

It was just after visiting hours ended one evening that the light went on over Mr. Callahan's door. The nurses were at the nurses' station doing their charts. "Oh, no," said Jill. "It's Mr. Whiner again. I can't stand going in there any more."

Rita stood up and sighed. "I'll get it this time," she said. She went into the room, Mr. Callahan was in his bed, propped up like a king with his five pillows strategically arranged all around him exactly like he always wanted.

"I coughed and I felt something pop," whined Mr. Callahan. "Maybe I broke a stitch," he added in his nasal droning voice.

"I doubt that, answered Rita with a trace of annoyance in her voice. "Mr. Callahan, you are fine. We just got you back to bed and you really have to try to relax and stop worrying so much. Watch some television for now, and we'll come in soon and get you ready for sleep."

Mr. Callahan didn't answer, but just turned his head. Rita left the room and went back to the nurses' station. Five minutes later the bell rang again. "I can't stand this any more," announced Rita. "It's your turn now, Tom."

Tom went into Mr. Callahan's room and went up to the bed. "Nobody listens to me," wailed Mr. Callahan in his high pitched grating voice. "Something popped in my stomach and now it feels wet," he stated.

Tom looked at Mr. Callahan's dressing. It seemed dry and intact. "Your dressing seems fine, Mr. Callahan," said Tom.

"Well, I don't care what it seems like," sniveled Mr. Callahan. "It feels weird."

Tom sighed out loud and thought to himself that it's not the dressing, but Mr. Whiner who is weird. But instead Tom said, "OK, Mr. Callahan. I'll look under the dressing and show you that everything is the way it should be. That way you will be satisfied that everything is OK."

"Good," said Mr. Callahan in his whiny voice.

Tom peeled back the tape and raised up the dressing, totally unprepared for what he found. There, right on the outside of Mr. Callahan's abdomen, were about eight inches of small intestine which had eviscerated right through the open abdominal wound. Obviously that is what Mr. Whiner felt crawling across his skin. It was his own intestines.

Tom had seen wounds open up before, but it was the first time he had seen a true evisceration. Somehow he managed to keep himself calm and collected, since all Mr. Whiner had to see was his nurse freak out. "Well, Mr. Callahan," said Tom quietly. "It seems you're right. Your stitches did open up. Now you need to lie here quietly while I call your doctor."

"Oh, I knew it," howled Mr. Whiner. "I just knew something horrible was going to happen to me. I can't look! I can't look!"

For once Tom was glad to agree with Mr. Whiner. "Close your eyes, then," said Tom. "and wait till I get back."

Tom walked out to the desk where Rita and Jill were still charting. "You'll never believe this one," Tom said with a great big grin. "Mr. Whiner has eviscerated and his bowels are hanging out."

"Yeah, sure," said Jill, without looking up.

"OK, don't believe me," answered Tom as he began to dial the page line to call the surgical resident.

It was only when Jill and Rita heard Tom tell the resident what had happened that they finally believed him. Then the three nurses went back to Mr. Callahan's bedside with lots of sterile dressings and normal saline. They took the old dressing off and covered the still pink and glistening intestines with the soaking wet compresses to keep everything from drying out. It was gross, but all three of them kept straight faces. Mr. Whiner kept his eyes shut and, thankfully, did the same with his mouth. He probably was too surprised that the nurses finally agreed with something he said.

Anyway, Mr. Callahan wound up going back to the operating room to have his intestines put back inside his abdomen where they belonged. And, somehow, the extent of his whining decreased sharply, perhaps due to the shock of what happened or maybe simply because the nurses began to listen to what he had to say. And, Mr. Callahan remained known as Mr. Whiner until the day he was discharged.

THE GOURMET MEAL

Jeffrey Kaplan had arrived in the emergency department complaining of abdominal pain. While giving a history to the triage nurse, he casually mentioned that he had eaten some things that probably "just didn't agree with him."

Questioned further, Jeffrey clarified what these "things" were. A set of keys, a bunch of bottle caps, a key chain, about twenty-five coins - all kinds, a few safety pins, and some broken glass. Why did he eat these things? Smiling knowingly, Jeffrey whispered that the voices told him to do it.

Jeffrey was taken off to x-ray for abdominal films, and sure enough, he was telling the truth -- and more. He had forgotten to mention the paper clips.

So, up to the floor he came to be observed. The doctors wanted to see what would come out naturally, since nothing had yet seemed to damage his gastrointestinal tract.

Jeffrey was a perfect patient. He was polite and friendly with a warm cheerful smile. "Those darned voices," laughed Jeffrey, "always seem to get me into trouble!" And so he was given laxatives and everyone waited for nature to call.

Nature called that night. And the next morning. And the next night. The nurses had specimen jars full of Jeffrey's meals. Just about everything came out, including the glass. He was transferred to the psychiatric unit where the mental health staff began to help Jeffrey deal with those voices.

At the end of his hospitalization, x-rays showed two remaining paper clips which were sitting harmlessly in the curve of his small intestine. Jeffrey and his paper clips left the hospital together.

DESSERT

Lorrie finished Mrs. O'Donnell's morning care late that day; in fact it was almost lunch time when the bath basin was finally put away. "Try to eat as much as you can, Mrs. O'Donnell," said Lorrie, as she set the sweet little old lady up with her first regular lunch tray. "You have to eat to get your strength back, and then you'll see how fast you'll start to feel better." Lorrie went out of the room and left Mrs. O'Donnell with her tray.

After about 20 minutes, Lorrie returned. "How'd you do, Mrs. O'Donnell?" cheerily asked Lorrie.

"Well, dear, I ate almost everything on the tray, but I couldn't quite finish this tea biscuit," Mr. O'Donnell answered. "It tastes a little funny."

"Uh, that's OK, Mrs. O'Donnell," said Lorrie as she quickly threw out the half eaten bar of Dial soap which had been left on the overbed table next to the tray. "I think you've eaten enough."

MEAT HOOKS

It was a good thing she was able to walk to the ambulance, since it was unlikely that they could have picked her up and put her on the stretcher. The last time she was weighed, she told them, she had passed the six hundred pound mark. And that was well over a year ago.

Now she could barely breathe. Oh, they gave her all kinds of diagnoses from plain old respiratory failure to the catch-all Pickwickian syndrome. The bottom line was that she was morbidly obese and her lungs just couldn't work any more.

After an hour in the emergency department, it was obvious that Shirley was going to stop breathing. It was time to intubate her before this turned into a full code. Surprisingly enough, the intubation was relatively easy. It was, however, a little harder to get a foley into her, but that mission was also accomplished. A tribute to the emergency room nurses, they said.

The staff of the ICU needed to get ready for their six hundred pound plus patient. Back then there were no Mega-beds, and it was obvious that Shirley would not fit into any kind of a regular one unless they left the side rails down. Of course, this was a no-no. Everyone who even thought of doing that immediately pictured her falling on the floor as she tried to turn. Forget that. Remember, a six hundred pound person is equal to four one hundred fifty pound people. It was also very likely that she weighed more than that.

An extra bed was brought up to the unit and the two were put together in the room, side by side. A maintenance man came up and installed a bracket to hold the two lowered middle side rails together. That worked great and it looked like a jumbo bed. Then the nurses laid two air mattresses and two egg crates on the bed and nobody could even tell there was a crack between the two mattresses. Once the bed was made up, it looked comfortable.

Shirley was finally wheeled up to the unit on a regular stretcher. The side rails, of course, were down and there were three people on each side of the stretcher acting just like trampoline spotters. Shirley was balanced right in the middle of the stretcher. She was then slid easily into the center of the big bed across the Smooth Mover sliding board. Piece of cake.

Shirley was a very lovely and gracious lady. Her family told the staff that she had always been overweight, but the massive weight gain had occurred over the past five years. At home she spent most of the time in a special recliner, and the family and visiting nurses gave her sponge baths right in the chair. She was able to walk to the bathroom and somehow could balance herself over the toilet.

Of course that was when she was still able to breathe, and needless to say the nurses were now were very thankful for that foley catheter.

Nobody could ask for a more pleasant and cooperative patient. She did as much for herself as she possibly could. Bath time, naturally, took several nurses and aides, since some had to hold up her huge arms and legs while others washed. It was not easy to get a washcloth into all of Shirley's cracks and crevices, but every day she was washed and creamed and lotioned. The nurses had to literally climb into the bed to take care of Shirley since she was right in the center of it, but she got great care.

It was obvious from day one that Shirley was not going to be weaned quickly from the ventilator. So she had a tracheostomy done right in the big bed in the same room. It was decided that it would be safer to do it that way than try to move her to an operating room. Shirley slid to the side of the bed and the trach was done under local anesthesia. Although the surgeon and the anesthesiologist worried about problems from having to cut through all that tissue to reach the trachea, everything went smoothly. Afterwards, Shirley was much more comfortable and was able to begin taking clear fluids by mouth.

Shirley's abdomen was absolutely huge. Even lying on her back it hung down below her knees. The weight of it had pushed her diaphragm up and out, and her lungs could no longer mechanically function. They called that big mound of tissue a panniculus, and described it as a big subcutaneous layer of fascia which was filled with fat cells.

After several conferences and many consults, it was decided that the best way to help Shirley breathe again was to get rid of that panniculus, so as to allow her lungs to move down to where they belonged in her chest. However, this was not exactly a simple matter. It was felt that the panniculus itself weighed several hundred pounds, and was not just filled with fat. There was blood and body fluid and everything else circulating through it. The tissue had to be drained first in order to dehydrate it as much as possible.

So this was the idea. Surgeons would insert several tongs into the panniculus. Then, over a period of a few days, they would hoist it up higher and higher so it would empty itself very slowly. If it took place too fast, they could throw her into pulmonary edema by dumping that huge volume of fluid back into her circulation. Well, the plan took shape. Shirley agreed to do whatever had to be done to get better.

The next morning "operation meat hook" began. A special reinforced bed frame was installed, just like the frames that the traction and overhead trapezes hang from. A pulley system was set up and three heavy tongs were inserted, under local anesthesia, deep into Shirley's abdomen. Then, just like skeletal traction, the tongs were tightened to lift the panniculus up. The plan was to increase the traction every eight hours so as to raise the abdominal hump higher and higher.

Poor Shirley. You can imagine what a sight that was. And, of course the whole hospital was buzzing with what was going on. Even with the curtain closed, somehow the word spread. It seemed that everyone knew about the lady hanging up by the meat hooks. Shirley tried to laugh about it. She was absolutely flat on her back. Her biggest problem was back care, since she had to lie flat on her back. Even with the trapeze to pull herself up on, it was very hard to lift enough for the nurses to get at her back. The hooks hurt her when she moved.

The surgery was scheduled for the third day. Obviously she was to be brought to the operating room, for this was to be a very big procedure. But, the evening before the planned surgery, Shirley developed chest pain, and it turned out to be a true heart attack. So, after all of this, the surgery had to be canceled since there was no way that any procedure could be done to a patient who had just infarcted. The panniculus was then lowered slowly, just the same way as it had been raised, and then the meat hooks were removed. The whole plan was canceled.

Shirley spent the next several months attached to her ventilator, drinking clear fluids, and loosing weight. After a while, she improved enough to breathe on her own. By the time Shirley left the hospital, she was about one hundred fifty pounds lighter. Maybe the heart attack was a warning that sometimes the safest way to do something is just to do nothing at all.

THE EYEBALL

He had been on that respirator for about four days now, long enough to have to start making some decisions. It didn't appear that Mr. Hanson was doing much in the way of breathing on his own, and so they needed to start to plan for what should come next.

Mr. Hanson had suffered some sort of a stroke and had been found on the floor after a period of close to twenty-four hours. His wife had been visiting her sister in another state, and she had called home and spoken with her husband the evening that she had arrived. Then the next night when she tried to reach him, nobody had answered the phone and the police had been called. Mr. Hanson was then found on the bathroom floor.

Now he lay in that hospital bed, responsive only to pain, and with a really poor prognosis. Mrs. Hanson stayed with him from morning to night, going home only to sleep. Each morning, when she arrived back at the hospital, Mrs. Hanson fully expected to find her husband wide awake and talking. She had been informed by the doctors and nurses just how serious the situation was but Mrs. Hanson refused to believe it. In fact, she said over and over again when someone began to talk about her husband's prognosis, "I don't want to hear that kind of talk. I won't listen to it. I know my husband is going to get better." And she would turn her back and walk away from whomever was doing the talking.

A week went by. Mr. Hanson still could barely breathe on his own. Plus, it seemed now that he was developing pneumonia. He was full of mucus and needed suctioning constantly. It was obvious that he needed to have a tracheostomy done, since it was just not good medicine to leave that tube in place much longer. The doctors and nurses tried to talk to Mrs. Hanson. They explained just what it meant to have a trach and how Mr. Hanson's mouth and throat and vocal cords were becoming more and more swollen and irritated by that big tube which went through his mouth and down into his trachea. They demonstrated how a trach works and how much more comfortable patients are once the procedure is performed. Mrs. Hanson said she would absolutely not allow it.

Then, two of the nurses, Louise and Emma, decided it might be more effective if Mrs. Hanson saw exactly what a tracheostomy looked like. They brought her into the room of a patient who was sitting up and feeding himself lunch, while breathing thorough his tracheostomy. He looked comfortable and alert and waved at the two nurses. Well, that should do it, thought Emma and Lousie.

Instead, when they stepped out in the corridor, Mrs. Hanson told them that the tracheostomy was probably the most horrible thing she had ever seen and that

101

"nobody would ever cut a hole in her husband's throat while she was alive to stop tit." So, that was that. At least for a while.

After two weeks, things were much worse. Even with all the antibiotics, suctioning, and respiratory treatments, Mr. Hanson's pneumonia had spread. By this time, he was breathing without the aid of the ventilator but still needed the endotracheal tube to maintain his airway. No matter which way the nurses positioned the tubing which came off the adapter, the air that Mr. Hanson exhaled still seemed to blow toward his face. And that infected vapor always managed to blow right into his eyes.

Later that week, Mr. Hanson's right eye started to look a little bloodshot. Then it became red. Cultures of the eye showed the same organisms that came from his lungs. Obviously the infection was spreading. Again, the doctors and nurses tried to talk Mrs. Hanson. Once more they stressed the importance of a tracheostomy, describing in detail what the back of his throat must look like by now, being compressed by that big endotracheal tube. They told her how the lung infection was spreading to his eye, and how this could be avoided by having the tracheostomy done. Absolutely not. Forget it. Mrs. Hanson would not even discuss this. What ever would be, would be, she said. Nobody was going to cut open her husband's throat.

Another week went by and Mr. Hanson's eye had turned bright green. Antibiotic drops and round the clock eye irrigation did nothing. Then the eye started to turn brown, and before long it started to shrivel up. After a month, the eyeball looked like a raisin. When the irrigation fluid touched it, it wiggled around, and Emma and Lousie were afraid it was going to dry out completely, come loose and fall out of the socket. By this time, the hospital had gone to court to try to become the guardian of Mr. Hanson and allow him to have the tracheostomy done. But the hospital lost and the courts allowed Mrs. Hanson to keep on making his medical decisions.

By this time, Mrs. Hanson had stopped talking about the time when her husband would wake up and be fine, but now she began to say that her main concern was to keep things as they were "until the time was right." What this meant, nobody was sure, but she said that there "would be a sign to show when it was time." This seemed a little spooky to the nurses, and everyone wondered what kind of a sign she was talking about.

One night, Louise had a nightmare that she was turning Mr. Hanson and his dried up eyeball fell out and rolled down the front of her uniform. She woke up in a cold sweat. That day, when she arrived at work, she learned that the little raisin that used to function as a seeing eye had indeed broken loose and had fallen out onto the sheets when Mr. Hanson was turned. But it just didn't seem like an eye at the time; it looked like a crusted piece of dirt or a dried bug, something that had never been part of a body.

The day after the eyeball fell out, Mr. Hanson finally died. He was found not breathing by the nursing staff, and by the time they tried to resuscitate him it was much too late. It was a funny things though. Mrs. Hanson seemed very relieved, since by this time the whole episode seemed to have turned into a war between the hospital and herself. That was the sign, she told them, smiling and nodding. It was the eyeball. The eye had no more use, so it had fallen out, and when Mr. Hanson's lungs stopped working completely, his heart stopped. And nobody had forced her to change that. The time was right and she had won.

SECTION FIVE

THE SPECIAL SIDE OF NURSING

JUST BEING THERE

Elaine had been to about a hundred codes and she figured that she'd seen about 500 people die during all her years as an ICU nurse. Why was this code bothering her so much? After all, the man was 77 years old. At that age, you figure, well, it's OK to die. So what was happening here?

The call for the cardiac arrest team had come over the public address system just as Elaine was getting on the elevator headed for the cafeteria. She had hesitated for a second or two, thinking that if she just kept going, she could make believe that she never heard the announcement. Her ICU colleagues would respond, assuming she was at lunch.

But she jumped out before the elevator doors closed. As it happened, the patient arrested while being transferred from the emergency department to the coronary care unit.

She arrived in the CCU to see the code team performing CPR on this man as they crashed through the doors of the unit. What really tugged at Elaine's heart was the look on his wife's face. She had been in the elevator with him as he took his last breath. Now she was leaning against the wall with her eyes closed, softly pleading, "Oh no, John. Oh, God, no!"

Elaine took the wife out to the waiting room. Mercifully, it was empty. They sat together on the long couch at the far end of the wall. Back in the unit, the rest of the team continued to go through the motions of the code protocol. Compress the chest. Breathe for him. Give drugs. Shock him. Elaine sat with the wife, just holding her tightly as she cried softly. She didn't say a word and neither did Elaine. It just seemed as if there was nothing to be said. About 10 minutes into the code, a resident came out to tell the wife that her husbands' condition was critical, but that everything possible was being done. Still the wife said nothing, just holding tighter to Elaine.

After another 10 minutes passed, the code was discontinued. A physician came out to tell the wife what she already knew. She responded only with the words, "Please let me see him."

Elaine escorted her into the room. The area had been straightened, and the body was covered with fresh, crisp linen. The wife leaned over her husband and started kissing his face. She never even noticed the tube sticking out of his mouth. "John, don't leave me," she cried softly. "I can't believe you're gone."

That's when it hit Elaine. She started to cry with the wife. They probably had been married for 50 years and had six kids and sixteen grandchildren. Just this morning they had probably eaten breakfast together, just as they had done so many times before. How was she going to eat breakfast without him tomorrow?

Elaine took a handful of tissues from the box she had given the wife and wiped her face. It was then that the wife turned to Elaine and looked into her eyes, seemingly noticing her for the first time. Finally, she spoke.

"I don't know what I would have done out there without you, dear," she said loudly and clearly. "It was as if you were my daughter, sitting with me that way. Thank you for making sure that I wasn't alone."

Elaine suddenly remembered what she had said those many years ago at her pre-admission interview for nursing school. She had been asked why she wanted to become a nurse. "To help people," she had answered. Today, she had helped someone, and she was very glad that she was a nurse.

"Just Being There," by Linda Strangio, RN, MA, CCRN is reprinted with permission of *The Nursing Spectrum*, New York/New Jersey Metro Edition, Vol. 5A, No. 20, p. NJ-6, October 4, 1993.

THE ANGEL

He was just a kid. A seventeen year old kid. But he was a special seventeen year old kid, one with inoperable brain cancer. The surgery was done as an emergency, since three days after the tumor had been found, he began to have uncontrollable seizures. Less than half of the tumor could be removed, and Jack could no longer speak or even swallow. And, his right side was paralyzed.

Jack spent the next three months in the surgical intensive care unit, while doctors and nurses tried everything they could to prolong his life. He remained wide awake, and smiled and nodded at everyone who went into his room. Through all the painful tubes and treatments, the suctioning, and the blood tests, Jack stayed strong.

Jack's family became part of the surgical ICU family. They had been so close before he got sick, and the illness seemed to make them even more so. His older sister Phyllis and his mother moved into his room and stayed there with him. With two cots pushed up against the wall, that was their home. Each morning they folded up the cots and spent the day taking care of Jack. They helped bathe him and tube feed him and lift him out of bed. For two hours each day, Phyllis and Mama left to go shower and do a few errands. They cooked for Jack's dad, who spent his days at work and his evenings at the hospital.

While he never really was stable enough to leave the ICU, he began to deteriorate one night. The next morning Jack arrested and was placed back on the ventilator. Testing showed Jack to be brain dead. After two days, the decision was made to discontinue life support and let Jack go.

It was a bright Saturday afternoon in August, just the type of day that Jack loved. At about two o'clock, the people started to arrive at the hospital. By two-thirty there must have been a hundred people lined up outside the ICU. Most of the junior class of Jack's high school were there, along with teachers, friends and neighbors. Everyone had been invited to come to say good-bye to Jack, a boy who was obviously loved by everyone who knew him.

Then one by one, each person filed into his room. Each one said good-bye, most tearfully, some with smiles. Some kissed him and told him how much they loved him and would miss him. The big strong boys came out with tears streaming down their cheeks and the girls came out crying softly. The nurses watched some of the boys kiss his bald head and heard them tell him they cared about him. Then it was the family's turn. All the relatives came in to see Jack one more time.

By the time they were ready to terminate the life support, there were close to one hundred fifty people in the unit. Everyone held hands as the chain of people formed a big circle from the door of Jack's room, through the unit, down the long corridor, and back again to Jack's doorway. Housekeepers, food service workers, nurses, pharmacists, and people from all over the hospital were all there as one. The two hospital chaplains led the group in the Lord's Prayer as other patients' visitors joined in. At that point, everyone except the immediate family was asked to leave.

Jack was pronounced legally dead and then one of the doctors and two of Jack's nurses went in and took the ventilator off Jack's traceostomy and turned off the alarms. It took about fifteen minutes for Jack's heart to stop. Then it was all over and Jack's parents, grandmother, and Phyllis finally left the hospital.

There is a story that as they were walking sadly out to their car, they looked up and saw a formation of two hundred white birds soaring together up to the sky, and those birds were the spirits of love of all those people who helped Jack die so peacefully and so beautifully. And, the one bird in front was the angel called Jack.

FALLEN LEAVES

The headaches had begun just two weeks earlier, and like most people, Jerry attributed them to nothing serious. After all, everyone gets headaches. It wasn't until they became unbearable that Jerry went to see his physician. An MRI showed the mass.

The day before he was 32, Jerry had his first craniotomy. The neurosurgeons found just what they expected -- a highly malignant and inoperable brain tumor. Two days later, when his brain suddenly and dangerously began to swell, Jerry returned to the operating room for more surgery.

In just a few short weeks, Jerry's life had turned upside down. His wife blamed herself, arguing that she should have made him call the doctor earlier. She was sure he could have been cured if the tumor was smaller and if it had been found when the headaches first began. The doctors told her that with this particular grade of tumor, Jerry could not have been cured surgically even if they had tried to remove it when it was the size of a pea. Jerry's wife still wasn't so sure.

The staff had hoped they could discharge Jerry home and bring him back daily for radiation therapy as an outpatient. Their plan was to try to shrink the remaining cancer and give Jerry some more time. But this was not to be.

The craniotomy performed to save Jerry's life had severely damaged part of his brain. He could not speak or move his right side. He couldn't swallow very well and his cough reflex was weak. So now Jerry needed to be tube fed and was respirator dependent. He remained awake, alert, and full of life. This once big strong construction worker was now helpless. He needed a tube to eat and a tube to breathe, and was incontinent. But, Jerry never showed signs of withdrawal or of giving up.

Jerry wanted to live. He spelled out words with his left hand on the big communications board. His wife and parents stayed with him and encouraged him. He never gave up. Each day for five weeks, Jerry went for radiation treatments. While the oncologists felt that therapy was keeping this virulent tumor from growing faster, the tumor was not shrinking. They warned that when the treatments were over, it was likely that the tumor would again take off and start to grow rapidly. But everyone stayed optimistic for Jerry's sake.

Carol became Jerry's favorite nurse, sitting with him and talking to him about the Giants football team. After all, they were both Giant fanatics. Jerry loved that. He also loved the fall, and this was October, his favorite time of year. Jerry's wife told Carol how he loved to be outside when the leaves were on the ground and the weather was crisp and cold. One of the notes he had written on the alphabet board was how he wished he could walk through the fallen leaves again.

After a few weeks, Jerry was weaned from the ventilator but still needed the tracheostomy. A gastrostomy was performed so that the nasogastric tube could be removed, and Jerry's indwelling catheter was replaced with an external one. But, Jerry was too sick to leave the step-down unit; he had developed pneumonia and needed to be suctioned very frequently. His buttocks became excoriated from frequent diarrhea and he lost a great deal of weight despite hyperalimenation. Jerry was getting weaker and he was almost at the end of his radiation therapy.

One sunny and cold Sunday in early November, Carol had an idea. She decided she was going to give Jerry one more chance to see those autumn leaves. The floor was quiet and the census was low. Carol, Debbie, and Pearl went to tell Jerry, who was up in the big soft chair ready to watch the Giant game. "Come on Jerry," announced Carol with a big grin. "We're going traveling."

Bundled under four blankets and with the portable oxygen tank and two IV poles trailing, the three nurses took Jerry out of the unit and down the back corridor toward the emergency department entrance. People stared at the strange looking group and at this skinny but smiling young man with a Giants cap on his head, almost completely bald from his radiation treatments.

They wheeled Jerry all the way down the ramp and out onto the sidewalk in front of the hospital. Carol ran down into the street and, scooping up a big pile of leaves, came back and dumped them all over Jerry. Jerry began to laugh and cry at the same time. It was as if they all knew this was his good-bye to the world outside of the hospital. And suddenly everything seemed okay.

When Jerry was put back to bed after the football game was over, he fell into a sound sleep. Within a week, Jerry became less and less responsive and more and more septic. At this time, the family felt that Jerry was ready to let go, and a DNR order was put on his chart. Jerry died in his sleep the next day, perhaps while having a beautiful dream about walking in the autumn leaves.

THE FAMILY

Martin Wellington was lucky. He wasn't killed when, in the process of trimming tree limbs, he fell 30 feet to the ground. He was admitted to the surgical intensive care unit with both legs broken, his thoracic spine fractured, and some minor lacerations and bruises. Though he could easily have ended up a paraplegic, he had no neurological damage. To stabilize his spinal injury, Martin was scheduled to undergo a long operative procedure. But Martin's biggest worry was not the impending surgery; it was his family.

The 21 year old Martin was married and the father of a three month old baby. The young family of three lived in a small furnished room. Martin's wife, Nancy, stayed home with their baby while Martin did day-to-day yard work. He had no insurance and their rent was due the day of the accident. Neither Martin nor Nancy had any; family. Now Nancy and the baby had no place to go. Plus, Nancy did not want to leave Martin's bedside and had no one to watch the baby.

The surgical ICU nurses had a conference and decided to "adopt" this young family. Martin was transferred to the large corner room in the ICU, and Nancy and the baby moved into Martin's room with him. That evening after work, one of the nurses drove her van to Nancy's rooming house and helped her pack up their few belongings. The crib was placed in the corner, and clothes and baby things were put in the unit's storeroom. The nurses set up an unofficial fund for the family, with each person contributing whatever they wanted to give, money or otherwise. Word quickly spread to the other two intensive care units. Before long Martin, Nancy, and the baby had a large extended family. A nice little savings account was building, too.

Some money was allocated for food and diapers and other personal needs. The nursing staff took turns bringing clothes home to wash, and Nancy used the shower in the nurses' lounge. She slept in a recliner in Martin's room. Although none of this was officially recognized by the hospital administration, everyone knew about it.

When it was time to transfer Martin to the orthopedic floor after about two weeks in the ICU, he was put in a private room and the family lived together on the fifth floor. The orthopedic nurses joined the "family" and the money and caring grew.

After a while, Martin was transferred to a rehabilitation center. By this time, Nancy had enough money to go back to live in a one-room apartment. The nurses helped her move.

This story has a very happy ending. Martin recovered and went back to work, this time in a supermarket. He also enrolled part time in a community college, where he is studying business. The baby is now a happy toddler with the biggest family of aunts and uncles anyone could hope for.

"The Family," by Linda Strangio, RN, MA, CCRN is reprinted with permission of *The Nursing Spectrum*, New York/New Jersey Metro Edition, Vol. 6A, No. 24, November 28, 1994.

RATSO

His name was Richard Rafferty, but they called him "Ratso." He was a regular in the hospital, both in the medical clinic and as an inpatient. When he had enough money, Ratso lived in a furnished room, but most of the time he lived on the streets.

He was only in his forties, but had the body of a much older man. Mr. Rafferty was a diabetic, and never seemed to be under any type of control. He had high blood pressure, very poor circulation, and multiple leg ulcers.

When Ratso got tired of being outside, he spent whatever dollars he had on bags of candy. He knew that would throw his diabetes off enough to earn him at least a week in the hospital. And, that would guarantee him a warm comfortable bed and three good meals a day. Ratso always was ready to leave again, because while he was in the hospital he couldn't smoke his cigarettes or drink his wine.

Beside the diabetes, Ratso also had gall stones. Since his dietary habits were not exactly conducive to managing gall bladder disease, some of his hospitalizations resulted from the times his gall bladder flared up and made him sick. Often Mr. Rafferty found himself in one of the intensive care units, rather than the general medical-surgical floors reserved for the "ward service" patients. Then his care was also given by the various medical and surgical specialists, rather than only the medical residents.

Lots of nurses resented Ratso. After all, often he was quite sick and really needed an ICU bed. When he finally had his gall bladder removed, he needed a Swan-Ganz catheter and even spent two days on a ventilator. But, the staff reasoned, if he took better care of himself he wouldn't be in this situation. Who paid his tremendous medical bills? They did, indirectly.

Mr. Rafferty could be very charming when he wanted something. He was quite manipulative with both the nurses and doctors, and most of the hospital staff just couldn't help liking him. Nobody actually felt sorry for Ratso, because somehow he never felt sorry for himself. Two of the nurses, Pat and Jane, became Ratso's friends. They always asked to take care of him when he was admitted, and when he visited the medical clinic, he sent them his regards. They understood Ratso, and if they overheard anyone talking about him, they put a stop to it.

People wondered why Ratso Rafferty didn't take care of himself. He didn't follow a diet, he didn't monitor his blood sugars, and he rarely took insulin. Ratso simply lived as he liked between the times he was sick. He did keep his clinic appointments, though. It was a social occasion for him, to visit all the people who cared for him and the many who cared about him.

One day Ratso Rafferty didn't show up for clinic. There was no phone number, of course. A few days later, Richard Rafferty was found dead in an unheated garage. He had a big half eaten bag of Doritos and his vial of insulin with him at the time.

Richard Rafferty was just one of the "Ratsos" out there on the street, one of the many who lived a lifestyle most of us don't understand. Of course, Mr. Rafferty was non-compliant. Of course, he couldn't do finger sticks to check his blood sugars. Of course, he couldn't follow a diabetic diet. No wonder he died. And, no wonder he had nurses like Pat and Jane to care about him.

HE DIDN'T DIE ALONE

Like too many others, he was just called John Doe.

The Mobile Intensive Care Unit brought him to the Emergency Department after finding the old man on the ground in front of the supermarket. He was unresponsive and barely breathing.

He had no identification, no wallet, no keys, and no papers of any kind. The only thing they found in his pockets were carefully clipped grocery coupons for orange juice and dog food. John Doe was intubated and admitted to the intensive care unit where he was placed on a ventilator. Nobody came to visit since nobody seemed to miss him or even know he was in the hospital. Social Service had nobody to contact. The police had no reports of a missing person who fit his description; in fact there were no phone calls made to the police department to inquire about anyone who even resembled him.

The police investigations showed nobody who knew about this man. Two of the supermarket employees who saw him on the ground that morning thought they might have seen him in the store a few times, but they remembered nothing else about him. He was just an old man.

The evening supervisor, Irene Stone, found herself spending her breaks at John Doe's bedside. She was worried, not so much about him, but was afraid there might be someone left at home. Maybe there was a bed-ridden wife who was unable to help herself or even get to the phone. Could it be that was why nobody called about him? Or maybe there was no phone. And what about those dog food coupons? Was there a poor little dog at home alone locked in the house with no food and nobody to take care of it? John Doe, himself, was in good hands and was receiving the best of care.

Irene spoke to the public relations department of the hospital. They called the various police precincts and the local newspapers daily. Nothing. No response. Finally, Irene called the newspapers herself and a reporter came out to the hospital to do a story on John Doe. They took a picture of him and printed it under the caption, *"Do You Know This Man?"* Even with the endotracheal tube in his mouth and the feeding tube in his nose, his face could be clearly seen. But, nobody called. How could a person, a human being, not be known by anyone?

After about two weeks, John Doe died. His body was sent to the morgue and the very next day the hospital received a call from the police department. An old lady from upstate had contacted them because her brother had not called her for a long time, and he didn't answer his phone. She told them he had no friends and little money and was in poor health. His sister was afraid something had happened and she wanted the police to check on him. When his picture was faxed to the police upstate, the lady had identified her brother, Raymond, as being the John Doe in the picture. To Irene's relief, there was no wife and there were no pets.

Raymond's body was finally buried. A week later, Irene received a letter from his sister, who apparently had been given a copy of the newspaper article describing Irene's attempts to find the family. The lady thanked Irene profusely, writing a beautiful letter about the kindness shown to a complete stranger. Irene responded, writing back that Raymond did not die alone, and that he was cared for by a nursing staff who treated him with kindness and dignity.

Perhaps Raymond died better than he lived -- surrounded by nurses who took a John Doe and made him a very special person, one who no longer lived alone and ate dog food. In death, Raymond had found the caring that was missing from his life.

THE GOOD SAMARITAN

Eileen only needed to stop for a couple of things that September afternoon. Just some bread, milk, and hamburger meat for supper. It had been a rough day and she couldn't wait to get home. Tonight was the night they would eat early and then she would get into bed and watch television. With any luck, she'd be asleep by ten o'clock.

It was quarter after four when Eileen finally got to the Grand Union. She was glad to see it wasn't very crowded, since that meant she would be home even earlier. Eileen chose the items she wanted and then, as she knew she would, started browsing up and down the aisles. Eileen liked this store. They always had everything in stock. She was just putting a bottle of shampoo in her shopping cart when she heard the bang.

It sounded like it came form the back of the store, by the dairy items, and Eileen assumed that a display had fallen over. Eileen continued her shopping, but then she heard shouting. Maybe there is a fight, thought Eileen, and so she made her way over to see what was going on.

As she rounded the corner of the store she saw a lady lying on the ground, having a grand mal seizure. The convulsion involved her entire body and it was as violent a seizure as she'd ever seen. Eileen had been a nurse on a medical unit for twenty-two years, and had seen a lot of seizures. And, this lady was blue.

Before Eileen could do anything, somebody grabbed her by the arm, screaming, "Here's a nurse!" How does he know I'm a nurse, thought Eileen, and then she remembered she was wearing her white uniform with her name pin. The man literally pushed her down on the floor next to the lady, screaming, "Do something!"

By this time, it seemed that the seizure was beginning to slow down, but the lady still had that horrible blue color. She wasn't breathing, since the seizures hadn't completely stopped. Oh, God, thought Eileen. I'm going to have to do mouth to mouth right here on the floor in this Grand Union. Crazily, she looked up and down the aisles for an ambu bag, which of course wasn't there. She didn't have to feel for a pulse since she could see the carotid artery pounding in the lady's neck. Oh, breathe, lady, she begged silently. Please take a breath. The lady stopped seizing and started to breathe.

As her color slowly came back, the lady's respirations became easy and even. But, she remained unconscious in her post-ictal state. Some man screamed at Eileen, "Why don't you do something? She's dying and you're just letting her die!"

Eileen couldn't help it. She screamed back at the man, "She's not dying, so shut up!"

A few minutes later the lady on the floor started moving and trying to sit up. Eileen talked quietly to her and put her big overstuffed pocketbook under the lady's head like a pillow until the ambulance came. All during the time, bystanders were asking her questions, and some of them were pretty stupid. "What is wrong with her? Was that a fit? My cousin had a fit like that once and he had a brain tumor. Do you think she has a brain tumor?"

It seemed like forever until the ambulance arrived, and when it did, the EMT's took over. Eileen told them what happened and then stood up and got out of the way. Suddenly it was like she was invisible. Nobody thanked her or even looked at her. She realized she was shaking all over, but all the attention was still on the lady and the ambulance crew. She walked slowly back to her shopping cart, paid at the express checkout, and got out of the store as fast as she could. When she finally got in her car, she sat there a while until she calmed down a bit. Then she slowly drove home.

Eileen had a hard time sleeping that night, let alone following her plans for a peaceful quiet evening. She felt angry, but she really didn't know why.

Morning report started the next day before she could tell any of the nurses what had happened. And, as luck would have it, the patient in room 220 was a patient brought in last night after having a seizure in the Grand Union supermarket. Oh, God, said Eileen to herself. It's my seizure lady. The night nurse said the patient had a big lump on the side of her head, which she got when she fell. That's her, all right, thought Eileen. She had felt it starting to swell when she put the lady's head on the pocketbook. Then Eileen told her story, and everyone starting laughing.

Right after report Eileen went in to see the lady, who was wide awake. It turned out she was a known epileptic who had stopped taking her medication because she felt fine and decided she didn't need it anymore. Eileen told the lady she had been in the Grand Union with her the day before and what had happened.

"You know I hate that store," the lady announced. "I usually go to the big Grand Union near me, but yesterday I decided to stop there. My Grand Union is wonderful, but that one is no good. I never can get a good parking space there, and I always have to wait on line, and something always goes wrong. I never should have gone there. Can you get me another cup of tea?"

Eileen walked out of the room to get the tea. She didn't know how to feel. Did she really expect the lady to thank her for helping her? Did she feel she deserved something? Eileen just shook her head and smiled. Oh, well, she sighed. Tonight she'd go to sleep early.

THE WEDDING

Calvin was a very sick man when he was admitted to the hospital. He had been getting progressively worse at home, and at the time of his admission he could walk only a few steps before stopping to rest. Calvin had been hospitalized often with bouts of congestive heart failure, and with each admission he had gotten sicker and sicker.

But, this time, Calvin desperately did not want to be sick and in the hospital. He just kept hoping that he would start to improve on his own. Calvin's only daughter, Joyce, was to be married and the wedding date was almost three weeks away when he was brought to the emergency department. This time Calvin was so close to death that the usual drugs and treatment did not help. Calvin was put on a ventilator and an intra-aortic balloon was inserted to help his weak heart. His prognosis was grim.

Calvin's daughter Joyce, idolized her father. It had just been the two of them since she was eight years old when her mother died of breast cancer. She did not want her father to die before he saw her married. But it seemed that Calvin would not live the three weeks till her wedding.

The morning after Calvin was admitted, Joyce came in to the coronary care unit. She went straight to the nurses' station and asked for a conference with the nursing staff. Joyce had a plan and she needed the help of the hospital family.

On Saturday, Diane, Calvin's primary nurse, gave him his morning care extra early. Calvin fell asleep right afterwards, just as he always did after the slightest exertion. A little while later, Diane came in to Calvin's bedside and gently woke him. "Calvin," said Diane, "this is going to be a very special day for you."

At that point Calvin realized that a crowd had gathered in the middle of the coronary care unit, but he had no idea what was going on. In walked the pastor of Calvin's church, and all of a sudden Calvin realized what was happening. Uncertain that Calvin would be able to come to the wedding, the wedding came to Calvin.

It was beautiful. Many of the nurses said later that it was the best wedding they had ever attended. The maid of honor and the best man were there and there were flowers and taped music. Joyce wore her white bridal gown and held her father's hand all through the ceremony. The bride and bridegroom both hugged and kissed Calvin when it was over, and everyone cried tears of happiness.

The nurse gathered up the remnants of the insides of all the hole punchers in the hospital, and the tiny colored circles were distributed in little medication cups to be thrown at the bridal party.

The happiness of that day did something for Calvin. He started to improve rapidly and was weaned from both the balloon pump and the ventilator. Calvin regained his strength quickly and before long he was discharged home. A week after that, on their planned wedding day, Calvin proudly walked his daughter Joyce down the aisle of their church. He never felt better.

"The Wedding," by Linda Strangio, RN, MA, CCRN si reprinted with permission of *The Nursing Spectrum*, New York/New Jersey Metro Edition, Vol. 6A, No. 13, June, 1994.

SNOW

It came up the coast right on schedule. They called it a nor'easter and it was not an unusual event in February. But as with all storms, a few miles to the east or west decided whether there would be rain, snow, or a mixture of both.

This time it was all snow -- more than a foot of it. The winds, along with the drifting snow, made for blizzard-like conditions. Many offices and schools were closed and most unnecessary events were canceled. The roads were almost impassable. The radio and TV stations were telling everyone to stay home.

The first flakes had begun about one o'clock that morning, and by six there were already several inches on the ground. The staffing sheets, however, had only a very few red lines through names. It was, actually, a bit less than on any average day. Nurses come to work.

The incoming day shift arrived. Most of the nurses were on time, and some even early. They had given themselves plenty of time to clean off their cars, shovel out, and drive slowly on the unplowed roads. Many of the nurses brought overnight bags so that they could have a fresh change of clothes if they had to spend the night. After all, by the time their shifts were over, there would be quite a bit more snow and ice on the streets and it was likely that the next shift would have a much harder time getting through. Nurses plan ahead.

Breakfast was free in the cafeteria that morning. That's the way things were done at that hospital, and probably at most others also. It's a way of saying thank you for the extra effort of coming to work.

The day shifts of all the units hurried the night shifts through their morning reports so that the night nurses could get out as soon as possible, before the snowstorm got worse. Nurses care about each other.

Snow days are usually good days in hospitals. Everything is less. Doctors make quick rounds, or simply call in to check on their patients. Depending on staffing in other departments, testing is somewhat limited, so patients do not have to be packed up and transported to as many places. Visiting is minimal.

So, except for emergency situations, the floors and units are much quieter. If the laundry is not fully staffed, beds may not be completely changed. But as long as the patients are clean and dry, that's OK. Meals may be late, but they get there, and the drugs and supplies come up too. The atmosphere is different. It's more relaxed, more cheerful. Nurses cope.

Even the patients respond. Almost everyone has his or her television on, and weather updates are announced at frequent intervals. Patients seem to be satisfied with the less frantic and disruptive routine of a busy hospital floor. It's almost as if it's a welcome change from the focus of sickness and worry.

Today was no exception. The administrators made rounds, greeting the staff and offering thanks and encouragement. The snow continued on and the forecasts were calling for no letup until after midnight. Now quite a few nurses began to call to say that there was no way they could get in. But that was OK because the day shift never expected to get out either. Nurses understand.

So, as always in situations like this, plans were made to get through the night. Extra beds were gotten ready in various areas of the hospital. Empty patient rooms, on-call areas, lounges --- you name it --- preparations were made to take care of the staff. It was obvious that on floors where no new nurses could arrive, the already present staff would have to stagger sleep times. Arrangements were made for nurses to take a few hours to nap and then come back to relieve the others so they could also get some rest. Nurses organize.

So, the evening came and went and the night shift began. The snow finally changed to flurries around one AM and ended completely by three. The next day shift knew they would have to make it in; after all, they understood that their colleagues had been working for twenty-four hours. The plows had been going all night and the nurses who called to say they were still snowed in knew they would get there even if they would be a little late. Nurses know.

By nine o'clock that next morning, all nurses who had been there left. Some of the new evening shift arrived five or six hours early, in order to relieve those they knew needed to go home to rest. Nobody had to ask. Nurses feel for each other.

By that night, all was back to normal. but the special atmosphere remained, and the memories of the day of that nor'easter strengthened the ties between nurse at that hospital and at hospitals everywhere. Nurses share.

ALONE

Mr. Gray was seventy years old. He had lost his wife six months earlier after caring for her during her terminal illness. They had few friends and no family, and lived only for each other. When Mrs. Gray had been diagnosed with widespread cancer, he felt as if his world were coming to an end. Mr. Gray was not in the best of health himself, but did not ever go to see his doctor. He decided that if he did so, he probably would learn he had the same disease as his wife. He vowed not to die as she was doing.

Living alone and continuing to feel sick all the time, Mr. gray decided it was time to go and join his wife. He wrote a suicide note to whomever would find him, and sat down on his living room couch with his hunting rifle. Putting the barrel into his mouth, he aimed up and back so that the bullet would shatter his brain and he would die instantly. However, as Mr. Gray pulled the trigger, the gun moved to the side. Instead of the bullet firing up into the brain, it instead shot off the left side of his face.

The bullet completely missed all the important areas of his head; it whizzed past the jugular vein and the carotid artery, as well as bypassing his trachea and thyroid gland. It did, however, leave Mr. Gray with a missing jaw and cheek and only half of his tongue. He didn't look very pretty, but he was very much alive. So, not only didn't Mr. Gray get his wish, but now he was grossly disfigured, unable to even swallow or speak.

It was heartbreaking to take care of this poor little man. He had the biggest and saddest brown eyes which just seemed to emphasize his helplessness. They say the eyes are the mirror of the mind, and Mr. Gray's mind portrayed a lonely soul who now had even less to live for. All the nurses fell in love with Mr. Gray. He was so kind and gentle and the symbol of everyone's father or grandfather. Julie, his primary nurse, became especially attached to him.

Mr. Gray did not make a smooth recovery. When the bullet blew half of Mr. Gray's mouth into the side of his face, it also brought all the contamination of the oral cavity into the sterile bones and soft tissue. Pockets of infection continued to recur in what was left of the side of his face. Both the maxilla and mandible were affected, and the bone infection was a very difficult problem to control. He required several trips back to surgery, and long periods of intravenous antibiotics.

Julie and the nursing staff "adopted" Mr. Gray. He was so sweet and loving to everyone. He stoically endured all the wound irrigations and packings, and learned to give himself his own tube feedings. The chaplains, the social workers, the dietitians, and the patient representatives all adored Mr. Gray and tried to anticipate all his needs. They made arrangements with his bank, and managed his financial and home responsibilities.

Through all this Mr. Gray continued to show his thanks by nodding his head and by softly patting the hands of all who cared for him. Slowly he got better and was ready for discharge. On the day he left the hospital, the nursing staff presented him with a gigantic greeting card signed by everyone, which told him how very special he was. Julie put him into a cab and made him promise to come back in a week or so to show them that he was doing all right. Mr. Gray, his eyes filled with tears, just nodded and patted her hand.

Nobody ever heard from Mr. Gray again. He never showed up for his follow-up appointments and his phone was disconnected. When one of the social workers was able to reach his landlord, she was told that he had moved away and had left no forwarding address.

This was a long time ago. Those who were part of the staff when Mr. Gray was a patient still think about him and wonder what ever happened. Did they make a difference? Julie would like to think so.

A TIME TO DIE

It happened right before their eyes and in just a split second, all of their lives were changed. Jamie broke his neck while diving at the beach.

Things were a lot different back then. There were no trauma centers and no "miracle drugs" to help prevent damage to injured spinal cords. Jamie was paralyzed permanently and forever, and he was just twenty-five years old.

Jamie had six brothers and sisters and a loving mother and father. The family was very religious and extremely close. All of them accepted what had happened as God's will, and decided to take what lay ahead just one day at a time.

Today, Jamie would have been put into a halo vest and gotten up in a chair just a few days after the accident. But then the treatment was very different. Jamie was strapped to a turning frame with tongs in his head, where he was to remain for twelve weeks. Every few hours, Jamie had to be sandwiched between the two boards and manually flipped over. Jamie could lie only on his stomach or his back, flat on the frame.

Of course Jamie was wide awake. But whether it was his strong faith or his wonderful family, Jamie never seemed afraid. And, he was never alone. The parents had decided that Jamie, a very popular young man, needed time to spend with his friends. He always spent evenings out with them, and so now those hours were designated to be off limits for the family. Only friends were allowed in the room.

The nursing staff loved this plan. Those kids were absolutely great with him. They sat around the frame and talked and joked with him, and when he was on his belly, there were always one or two of the boys lying on the floor face up, talking to Jamie about everything that was going on in the world. They read the sports section of the newspaper out loud and listened to music with him. Anyone who passed that room never forgot the sight of a bunch of kids laughing and joking with another kid who just happened to lying on some weird contraption hooked up to a bunch of tubes and a respirator.

Jamie couldn't talk but he sure could mouth words and make his feelings known. He had long "discussions" with his family and friends about his physical condition and what he wanted for the future. Jamie also had long talks with his priest. He believed very strongly that life did not end with physical dying, and he was very certain that there was a beautiful hereafter. Even though he was so young, Jamie honestly and truly was not afraid to die. He felt that if death was meant to be, he didn't want to prolong the dying process. Even back then when there were no living wills or advanced directives, Jamie certainly made his wishes known.

After almost two months on the frame, complications set in. Within a short time, Jamie developed pneumonia and was full of secretions. He needed to be suctioned all the time and ran high fevers. Jamie was miserable. The antibiotics did not seem to make any headway against the infection and several areas in the lungs began to consolidate. Everyone knew that this was a real turning point.

One afternoon, Jamie developed severe respiratory distress. A portable x-ray showed a complete collapse of the right lung, which indicated the immediate need for a chest tube. Jamie looked straight at his doctors and nurses and clearly mouthed two word. No. Enough.

The doctors explained to Jamie what would happen if the tube wasn't put in. They described how the other lung and the trachea would start to move over to the side of the chest where the collapsed lung was, and how even with the respirator he would no longer be able to breathe at all. And, most importantly, they told him that then he would most certainly die.

Jamie smiled. He told the doctors that he understood all of this, and he still didn't want any more tubes. If that meant he would die, so be it. Jamie's parents smiled through their tears. There is a time for everything, they said, and also a time for death.

As the evening wore on, Jamie's breathing became more and more labored. He began to drift off to sleep, waking up only when he was suctioned. When he was awake he smiled peacefully at his family and best friend who stood around the bedside together. "We love you Jamie," each one called to him. "It's OK to let go and go to sleep." After a while Jamie stopped responding to the suction catheter and soon after that he fell into a deep coma. Jamie died peacefully, in a room filled with love.

There was a line two blocks long to get into the funeral home to pay respects to Jamie. Lots of the nursing staff went to the wake, since, after spending so long with someone like Jamie, they knew how very special he was. Although it would be very hard to conceive of how someone so young and so full of life could be so ready to accept death, it seemed easy to understand in this case. Jamie and his family truly believed that death was simply a natural part of life, something beautiful and peaceful.

The family donated a plaque, dedicated to the nurses of that unit who gave Jamie the dignity and grace to live and die the way he wished. And to this day, a little bit of Jamie's soul still remains to remind people just what life and love is all about.

SECTION SIX

AND MORE

PLAGUE

Chris was a petite blond nurse, only about 25 years old. She had curly hair and bright eyes. Always smiling, she was what other nurses called a "real nurse." Chris loved her job, adored her patients, and was happiest when she was at the bedside taking care of them. She did all the little extras that made her patients feel special.

She spent time combing her patients' hair, helped them rinse their dry mouths several times each shift, and made sure all her men patients were shaved. When Chris went grocery shopping, she always picked up stuff like hair spray, deodorant, perfumed talcum powder, and toothpaste to bring to work for patients who needed it. Chris never forgot that under all the tubes and wires there were real people. All the patients loved Chris.

Her first attack of bronchitis lasted a long time. She really felt sick, but only missed a day of work because she knew how hard it was on her co-workers when someone takes time off. Like the other nurses, Chris diagnosed herself by her symptoms and treated herself. Cough medicine, Tylenol, Nyquil -- the usual stuff. After a while, she felt better.

Then the cough came back, and this time it was worse. Her glands were swollen and she developed a fever. After two days of this, she did go to see a doctor and was given antibiotics. The coughing was awful and he told her that she might need to be hospitalized if she didn't improve, but Chris just stayed home in bed. She didn't want to be a patient.

Chris had lots of friends and they took turns calling and checking on her. She didn't get better right away, but at least she got no worse. It really was weird that Chris should be sick like this, everyone thought. She was usually so healthy -- she never even caught colds. Chris missed a week of work.

Chris and her friend Linda were saying good-bye at the end of the shift the first day that Chris was back to work when Linda took a long hard look at her. She looked absolutely exhausted. She had lost weight and her eyes just looked funny. Linda realized that Chris' hair had gotten very thin; she could see patches of her scalp. And, she was coughing again. Suddenly she knew what was wrong with Chris. Chris had AIDS and Linda wanted to vomit.

Two days later, they got the call. Chris was in the emergency department with an overwhelming pneumonia. She was critical.

They admitted Chris to her own intensive care unit. She was put on a respirator that night and before they put the tube down her throat, Chris tearfully made all of her friends promise that they would keep her heavily sedated. They gave Chris a few minutes alone with her parents first while she could still speak, and it was then that Chris told them that her ex-boyfriend was HIV positive. They all cried together. Five days later, Chris died.

KATHLEEN

They were just a couple of teenagers out joy riding. Eighteen and nineteen years old, they were still kids. But when the car hit that pole, that was the end of everything.

Richard had his seat belt on and he got away with just a couple of broken bones. But Kathleen was thrown through the front window and came close to dying right there on that street. The police estimated that they were going close to eighty miles an hour at the time of the accident, and most of the bones in Kathleen's face were shattered.

This once beautiful girl with the long blond hair no longer had any shape to her face. When some of the swelling finally started to subside, you couldn't really tell that she had a nose any more. Even after all the surgery, she was almost unrecognizable. Parts of her face had been torn away. She had suffered such damage to her eyes that she was totally blind.

Kathleen's and Richard's families had been feuding for years. It had started when they were little kids, and as they grew up and started to like each other, the fighting escalated. Kathleen's father had threatened to kill Richard if he ever saw Richard near Kathleen. Maybe that's one of the reasons they started going out together. You know how kids are.

After the accident, there were real problems. The hospital had to station security officers by each of their rooms because of all the threats. The day Richard was discharged, the hospital received a bomb threat that just about everyone believed came from his family.

Kathleen was awake. She knew she had been terribly hurt and of course she knew she was blind. Her mother came to see her, but her father refused to come. Maybe it was because he couldn't stand to see her like that, or maybe it was because he had followed through on his threat to disown her if she ever saw Richard again. Kathleen had episodes when she would become very agitated and almost frantic. Since she had a tracheostomy and couldn't speak, it was really hard to tell if she was confused during those times or just beside herself with terror. When Donna, her primary nurse, sat with her and spoke to her she settled down for a while. But then it started up all over again.

Richard couldn't visit her. Her family absolutely forbade it. They blamed him for Kathleen's injuries. Her uncles had called his house and said they would kill him if he ever tried to see her again. It was a horrible situation. All the nurses could tell her was that Richard was OK and he was home. Nobody really knew what she understood or even if she was wondering about him. Both her arms were broken, so Donna couldn't even attempt to have her write. And, she signaled "yes" to every question.

A month passed and Kathleen more or less stabilized. She was off the ventilator, but still had her tracheostomy. She was indeed permanently blind. Kathleen still had frequent episodes when she would become wild and try to pull out all her tubes. If she pulled out the trach tube, everyone knew she could suffocate. She had some infection still remaining in her neck which made the swelling there even more dangerous. Her hands were always kept tied.

Well, Kathleen was finally transferred out of the ICU to a room on a regular floor, directly across from the nurses' station. Donna was working evenings one day when she heard the cardiac arrest code called. It was for Kathleen's room. Donna ran up the two flights of stairs and down the corridor to the next building. When she got to the room, all she saw was blood. CPR was in progress, but Donna knew right away it was no use. Kathleen's carotid artery had eroded and blown out. Donna stepped back into the hall and waited until it was all over.

When everyone had left the room, Donna went in. Kathleen's beautiful long blond hair was matted with blood and clots. Her big blind wide eyes were coated with blood. You could hardly see them. Donna tried not to think of what happened when Kathleen's carotid artery blew, when she couldn't call out for help. Blood had spewn down her trachea and she had choked to death on it. And, her hands were tied. She couldn't even bang on the side rail or put her hands up to her throat. Donna went into the bathroom and vomited.

For weeks after that, Donna had nightmares. She never talked to anyone about how she had found Kathleen and about her recurrent vision of the way she had died. In time, the memory did begin to fade and it became a little easier to think about Kathleen. But, the hurting feeling never did go completely away. It probably never will.

THE PUSSY CAT

He came up from the emergency room accompanied by a policeman. Justin had been caught shoplifting, and when the store manager chased him out of the store, Justin had fallen on the ice. Besides his broken wrist, Justin banged his head and had been unconscious for a few minutes. He needed to be admitted overnight just to make sure there was nothing more serious than a mild concussion.

Justin was very apologetic. He was sorry for the inconvenience he had caused and for the bother to the nurses and doctors. Years ago he had also been arrested for shoplifting, but that was his only police record. He just wanted those cigarettes and didn't have the money. He asked the policeman to please apologize for him to the store manager. He told everyone how embarrassed he was and that when he was able, he would go back to the store to apologize in person.

Justin was the world's most polite patient. When his dinner tray arrived, he thanked the dietary aide profusely and told her how delicious everything looked. When the housekeeper came in to empty his wastebasket, he told her how clean everything was. He introduced himself to his roommate, Mr. Silver, and told him that if he needed anything, he would be glad to help. What a sweet man, everyone said. What a shame he had to be under police guard like a common criminal.

Marilou was Justin's nurse. When she came in to take his blood pressure, he thanked her for all her time. What a gentleman he was, everyone said. Marilou felt so sorry for Justin. He had big brown eyes and he seemed so sad. She didn't ask him, but she assumed he didn't have a real family or anybody who cared about him. He wasn't a real thief, she decided. If people walked past his room and saw the uniformed policeman outside, they would think that a real bad guy was inside. That wasn't fair. Justin wasn't bad.

Now this was a small town with a very small police force. Keeping a policeman at the bedside to baby-sit for a shoplifter was really a hardship, as well as an expense for the town. When the lieutenant stopped by on his rounds, the nurses asked if it was really necessary to have this poor soul guarded as if he were some kind of a murderer or something. "Justin is a pussycat," Marilou told the lieutenant. "Why don't you leave him here overnight and you can take him to the police station in the morning. He'll be good. He's so sweet."

For whatever reason, the decision was made to take the police guard away and put him back on patrol. "OK," said the lieutenant. "The pussycat's all yours for tonight. We'll see him in the morning." Justin thanked the policeman sincerely for their time and compassion. He assured them that when he was discharged the next morning, he would take full responsibility for his actions and he promised that he would give the nurses no trouble. Everyone was satisfied.

Marilou went to give out her medications. Fifteen minutes later, she walked past Justin's room. She looked in and saw both beds empty. Both of these men can't be in the bathroom at the same time, she thought uneasily. "Justin," Marilou called out. No answer. She knocked on the bathroom door and the other patient came out. "Where's Justin?" she asked.

"He was in bed watching television when I went into the bathroom." said the man. His eyes went to the open drawer of his bedside stand and his open closet door. "Uh, oh," said Mr. Silver. Not only was Justin gone, but so was Mr. Silver's wallet, wristwatch, and overcoat. The pussycat had escaped.

"Talk about using nursing judgment," moaned Marilou as she went out to call hospital security, her supervisor and the police. "I'll never live this one down."

ANEURYSM

She was at home vacuuming when she first felt the explosion in her head. The next thing she remembered, and not very clearly at that, she was in the hospital. The CT scan showed a big intracerebral bleed. A few days later the angiogram confirmed the ruptured aneurysm.

Back then there was no rush to operate, since all subarachnoid hemorrhages were treated with two full weeks of rest, allowing for any intravascular spasm to subside. So, Lorraine was admitted to the step-down unit to do nothing but stay in bed and rest, waiting for the time she could go to the operating room.

After a few days the headache began to subside, and Lorraine felt better. She was a great patient, and did everything she was supposed to do. She was funny and friendly and optimistic. All the nurses were able to relate to her, since she was about thirty years old and that was the average age of the nursing staff. Lorraine had a great sense of humor, and one of the things the nurses remembered most about her was her boisterous laugh. In fact, she had to be warned not too laugh too hard. That aneurysm had to stay sealed off.

Lorraine was a lesbian, and back then not too many homosexuals were "out of the closet." But Lorraine wasn't ashamed of her lifestyle and she was proud to show off her girlfriend. Lorraine's girlfriend was as bubbly and outgoing as she was. They did nutty things to keep everyone laughing. Lorraine kept an unrolled condom attached to the top of her IV pole. She called it her "conversation piece," and she loved shocking people who stopped by. The clergy and patient representatives got a big kick out of it.

Everyone was anxious for the surgery to take place. Lorraine wanted to get that "dumb thing clipped so I can go on with my life." After two weeks, the repeat angiogram showed no spasm and the operation was scheduled for that week. Nobody dreaded the surgery; in fact, it was looked forward to as the time that meant Lorraine could go back to being Lorraine.

On the morning of the surgery, Lorraine was wheeled to the operating room with a parade of well-wishers following her. The condom was attached to the portable IV pole, since Lorraine said she "wanted to be sure the operating room staff was wide awake." There was no doubt that she'd do great.

Six hours later, the surgery was called a great success. The aneurysm was clipped and Lorraine was awake in the recovery room. It couldn't have gone better. The next morning when the day shift came in, Lorraine was sitting up in bed. "Piece of cake," she said. "I'm ready to go home."

Those were the last words she ever said. Somehow, the artery went into spasm and cut off the blood supply to Lorraine's brain. In an hour she was dead.

In the years that followed many new advances were made in the treatment of patients with leaking or ruptured aneurysms. Early surgery and drug therapy help to prevent the dreaded vascular spasm which killed Lorraine. The nurses who knew Lorraine still think of the lady with the condom on her IV pole each time a subarachnoid hemorrhage patient is admitted. And they smile.

THEM

Marilyn saw his name in the obituary column. Richard Columbus. It was a funny kind of name, sort of dignified. You would expect a person named Richard Columbus to be just like his name. Very proper, and even maybe a little bit stuffy.

She remembered the first time she met him. He had just been admitted to the telemetry floor with a TIA. He had been at work as an executive in a big computer firm when his right arm and leg became numb. Then he began to have trouble speaking. He had probably scared his employees to death. They called an ambulance and he was brought to the hospital. By the time he arrived, he was pretty close to being OK again. He had just a little bit of residual weakness and a hint of slurred speech. An hour later all those symptoms were gone and Mr. Columbus wanted to go home. In fact, he wanted to go back to work.

Of course he was not advised to do that. Told this could be signs of an impending stroke, he decided to stay and have the tests the doctors wanted. A waste of money, though, Mr. Columbus announced. But, to make his wife happy, he followed orders. He'd stay overnight and then he was out of there. That was the deal he made. One night. Tests. And then home. He had too much to do. So, since it was six o'clock in the evening by then, the tests were ordered to be done the next morning. The usual tests were ordered -- echocardiogram, carotid Doppler ultrasound, etc. Nothing very exciting.

The next morning, when the day nurse made her first rounds, she found Richard Columbus in bed, incontinent of urine. He was babbling softly to himself and flailing around weakly with his left hand. His entire right side was flaccid. Mr. Columbus did not respond appropriately to verbal stimuli; in fact, he didn't seem to know anyone was speaking to him. Mr. Columbus had had a major stroke.

For the next five days, Richard Columbus continuously deteriorated. The CT scan showed his stroke had extended. Now Mr. Columbus no longer babbled. He was still; the only noise made was that of his breathing, which now was becoming more and more labored.

After much conversation with his family, the decision was made not to resuscitate him. Mr. Columbus would never want to live out his last days on a respirator in a condition such as that. The very next afternoon, Mr. Columbus died quietly and peacefully in his sleep, probably never having known what happened to him.

During those last few days of his life, Richard Columbus had become one of "them." He had crossed the line between a functioning rational human being and confused agitated patient.

This man had become what is known as a GOMER. Short for "Get Out of My Emergency Room," a GOMER is known in all hospitals as something of a "non-person." "They" are different than "us." After all, Mr. Columbus was restless and irrational, and was unable to respond to us. That's not the way human beings are supposed to be, is it? Only the non-people act like that, so Richard Columbus had become a non-person. Maybe it's easier for nurses to label these sick people and make them one group. Maybe that's why we do it. Maybe that's how we cope with what we have to deal with.

When Marilyn read about Richard Columbus in the obituary, she learned about his life. Where he went to school. What honors he had earned. His home. His family. His career. His clubs and organizations. He really was a person, this Richard Columbus. And, Marilyn then was able to bring Mr. Columbus back across that line, to change him from one of "them," back to one of "us."

Whether we like to admit it or not, there will be many other Richard Columbuses, other people who we turn into non-people. And, maybe we need to forgive ourselves when we realize what we do. For some of us, this may be the only way to accept what has happened to this human being. After all, it could never happen to us.

Could it?

I NOW PRONOUNCE YOU .... *??*

It seemed that she had been dying for a very long time. Too long. Nobody should have to go through that. Not the family, not the friends, and most of all, not the patient. It wasn't fair.

Four years earlier, Mrs. Bartholemew had been diagnosed with ALS, better known as Lou Gehrig's Disease. She had managed pretty well, up until a year ago when she had begun to really go downhill. Mrs. Bartholemew was seventy-two years old.

Six months ago she had become completely paralyzed and respirator dependent. It wouldn't be long now, the family was told. Her wishes were followed and she was made a "no-code." Plenty of people who are on respirators die at home these days, but not back then. Mrs. Bartholemew had to live in the hospital.

Finally, Mrs. Bartholemew went into a coma. Until then she had been able to raise her eyebrows and grimace when she wanted something, but now she was totally unresponsive. The entire family stayed around the bedside, keeping vigil. Even though they probably wanted this nightmare to be over, they still were afraid of the moment of death. That was very clear.

Mary Jane was Mrs. Bartholemew's nurse that evening. She went into her room to do a routine vital sign check. The family was there, crying and pacing around the room. The bellows on the spirometer went up and down with its preset volume. Twelve breaths per minute. Mrs. Bartholemew's eyes had been covered with moist patches to protect them from drying out. She looked dead, but she had looked that way for two days now.

Mary Jane picked up Mrs. Bartholemew's hand to check her pulse. Uh, oh, she said to herself. No pulse. She's dead. The family stared at Mary Jane, who was making believe she was counting the rate but instead was trying to figure out how to break the news to them. She knew she couldn't lie, but she also knew that when they found out Mrs. Bartholemew had died there was going to be a major scene.

Mary Jane took a deep breath and braced herself. "She's gone, I'm afraid," said Mary Jane softly.

"What did you say?" said Mrs. Bartholemew's daughter, with absolute terror in her eyes.

"Your mom has passed away," said Mary Jane gently. "I'm so very sorry."

The four people in the room started to scream as one. The two daughters threw themselves on top of the patient, crying out for their mother not to leave them. It was very emotional, to say the least. After a few minutes, Mary Jane got them to calm down a bit and maybe start to realize that what they had been both wanting yet fearing had happened. It was finally over.

Leaving the room to get the resident to pronounce Mrs. Bartholemew, Mary Jane heaved a sigh of relief. Most of the nurses had dreaded being there at the time of death, since they had anticipated what would happen. Well, that was that.

Mary Jane went up to her friend, Carolyn, who was working with her that evening. "Well," she said, "Mrs. Bartholemew finally died. I told the family all by myself cause I couldn't do it any other way. They acted just like we all thought, but they are better now. I'm glad that's over." Then Mary Jane paged the resident while Carolyn went into the room to get Mrs. Bartholemew's belongings together.

The family was seated across from the bed, crying softly but obviously much calmer then they had been. It seemed that relief was beginning to set in. Carolyn looked at Mrs. Bartholemew, who of course was still on the respirator since she hadn't been pronounced dead yet. The first thing she noticed was the carotid pulse. It was so strong that Carolyn could see it pounding from across the room. Quite obviously, Mrs. Bartholemew was far from dead, and with a pulse that strong she most likely had a pretty decent blood pressure too. "Uh, excuse me," mumbled Carolyn, as she turned back and walked slowly out of the room.

As soon as she got away from the doorway, Carolyn started to run. She got to the nurses' station just as Mary Jane was beginning to speak to the resident to tell him about the death. "Hang up," said Carolyn.

"What's wrong?" asked Mary Jane.

"I'll tell you what's wrong," frantically whispered Carolyn. "She's not dead. Now what do we say to the family? 'Oh, we made a mistake; she's not dead after all. Sorry, but she's still alive.' Oh, I'll kill you for this one, Mary Jane!"

"Oh, my god," moaned Mary Jane. "What are we going to do now?" They looked at each other and started to laugh from nervousness. Then Mary Jane walked slowly back into the room. The family just stared at her while she went back over and took the patient's blood pressure. Sure enough, it was one hundred over sixty. Mary Jane listened to the heart rate with her stethoscope. About eighty per minute. Mary Jane cleared her throat and turned toward the family.

"Something has changed with Mrs. Bartholemew's condition," she stated matter of factly. She now has a heart rate. Obviously when I checked her pulse before it was too faint to feel. But, it is there and she has not yet died." The family just stared at Mary Jane, who expected them to start screaming at her. Instead they jumped up and started grabbing each other and yelling, "Thank God! She's alive!"

Mary Jane left the room, telling herself that even if Mrs. Bartholemew really died later on that shift, she was not going to tell them. They'd never know, and she'd just leave her until the next shift found her.

That didn't happen though. Mrs. Bartholemew lived another three weeks, and died one night when no family was present and when Mary Jane was away on vacation. When it finally happened, it was quite uneventful, possibly since as far as the family was concerned, the main event had already taken place three weeks before.

TEAMWORK

It was a rare disorder, but he developed a type of gangrene just in his perineal area. It wasn't very bad at the beginning and only some minor debridement was done.

The gangrene began to spread, so Charles was returned to the operating room for more surgery. This time the surgery was much more involved. In fact, Charles' penis had to be "degloved," leaving it with no skin at all. His scrotum was removed, but the testicles were left in place. The perennial wound was left open.

Charles was in considerable pain, even with all the analgesics. The wound care was extensive and time consuming, and since his bottom had no skin to cover it, he lay on wet dressings and linens most of the time. As fast as the nurses changed them, his open body oozed fluids and saturated everything.

Despite all the antibiotics and fluids, the infection spread. Within two days, a white line of demarcation could be seen down both of Charles' thighs, up in front to his umbilicus, and around both sides midway up his back. The only hope for Charles was to return to the operating room again.

This surgery was much more radical. All of the skin and subcutaneous tissue was removed from Charles' thighs, perineum, sides, front and back, all the way up to his chest. His testicles were removed. Like a massive third degree burn, he was wide open.

There couldn't be more of a nursing challenge. Three times a day, all the packings and dressings had to be removed, and these were soaked not only with body fluids, but with foul-smelling purulent drainage. Then the areas needed to be irrigated and repacked. Certain areas needed to be covered with ointments and creams, and the whole procedure took about three hours. Charles was on a special bed, but even so it took four people to hold him over while the treatments were done. Ideally, he belonged in a burn unit, but with his overwhelming infection that was the last place he could be transferred to.

The nurses found that only a strong morphine IV drip could control Charles' pain. By this time Charles had developed septic shock and was on a ventilator, but the fear in his eyes when he was awakened for the dressings was horrible. Everyone felt these agonizing treatments were hopeless anyway, since Charles was going to die. Nobody wanted to hurt him anymore.

Charles received volumes of IV fluids and blood transfusions to try to keep up with the massive fluid losses suffered. His clotting factors were being depleted, and he was beginning to bleed from everywhere. The pigskin grafts placed over some of the surgical sites needed to be constantly replaced, since they seemed to lift up and wash away when the body fluids seeped out.

Most of the doctors felt it was time to stop. Charles needed to be kept comfortable until he died. The nurses agreed. The family agreed.

But, then a patient care conference was held with the family present, and one of the doctors honestly told the family that he still felt that Charles had a five percent chance to live. Now Charles had been a military man for all of his life, and he always was a fighter. The family decided to give Charles that small chance, since they felt that if he were awake enough to talk he would want to accept that challenge. In addition, the family learned that the strong morphine drip might be adding to his dangerously low blood pressure, and so they asked to have the medication stopped.

It was terribly frustrating to the nurses who spent so many hours with this poor man. But Charles' family felt that this hospital had basically given up on Charles, and if he was to make it, they needed to transfer him to another facility where everyone would give him one hundred percent of themselves to save him.

After many conferences and consults and phone calls, arrangements were made to transfer Charles. At this point, the nurses honestly were glad to see him go. It was as if they were torturing a dying man here and nobody wanted to do it anymore.

Two of the ICU nurses and a respiratory therapist went with Charles in the ambulance. Charles, with no skin to keep him warm, was transferred under ten blankets. The family signed the "against medical advice" form, adding in writing that they knew Charles was being transferred while in shock and bleeding profusely. One of the things which stood out in the mind of one of the nurses was the fact that the ambulance had to wait in a long line at the toll booth to pay the thirty-five cents, while Charles was on the verge of dying right then and there. But they got him there.

That started a daily report between the ICU nurses of both hospitals, a routine that lasted for two months. You see, Charles did not die. By the end of that week he seemed to turn around and start to improve. The grafting continued and the dressings and packings became less and less and the infection slowed down and gradually became under control. Charles became increasingly alert, and he was weaned off the respirator.

Two months after that, Charles was discharged. It would be easy to feel that the first hospital failed Charles, that the staff almost let him die. But, surprisingly, nobody felt that way. The nurses worked so hard and gave so much to Charles, but then decided it was time to step back and let others take over. And, the feeling from the other hospital's ICU nurses was remarkably the same. It was as if nurses just understand these things. It was a team, even if the team was split between two hospitals.

Nine months after Charles' discharge, he was admitted to a surgical floor at the first hospital for a minor revision of part of his weakened abdominal wall. The ICU nurses went up to see him and almost nobody recognized him. He looked great. Charles remembered nothing, of course, but he said he knew that if it wasn't for these nurses doing all they did those first few weeks, he was sure he would be dead.

So, was this a nursing failure? Absolutely not. It was a collaboration of skills and caring, a show of togetherness which resulted in a very happy ending.

SADNESS

Mary Ann had always been a shy girl. She had no dates and very few friends. Not very pretty and never a good student, Mary Ann had done very poorly during her junior year in high school. She was attending summer school to make up her course, but was doing even worse this time around. According to Mary Ann, her parents were constantly on her back telling her she was stupid and would never get into college.

She was receiving counseling, but that didn't seem to have any type of effect on her. She felt hopeless and helpless and wanted out. Mary Ann was admitted to the medical intensive care unit after having ingested an overdose of drugs which had been prescribed to help with her depression. This was the only answer, Mary Ann told the admitting staff. She couldn't cope with the world anymore.

Plans were made to move Mary Ann to the mental health unit in the morning, just as soon as everyone was sure that the antidepressants had not affected her heart. Her cardiac rhythm needed to be observed overnight, and so she was to spend the night in the ICU. She was placed on suicide precautions, checked very frequently, and not allowed to have any sharp items at her bedside. It was all very routine. After all, Mary Ann was just one of several attempted suicides admitted that week.

Mary Ann did whatever was asked of her. She said very little, was extremely polite and cooperative, and just lay quietly in her bed. It seemed, in fact, as if Mary Ann had just given up. Jackie and Corinne felt sad when they were in the room with Mary Ann; she seemed to believe that she wasn't worthy of anything good. It was even worse when Mary Ann's parents arrived. They gave the impression that once again she had disappointed them. Now, to add to everything else she had done, she had embarrassed them and put them through this ordeal.

Visiting hours ended and her parents left. Mary Ann's heart rhythm remained stable and she knew that she would be leaving the unit the next morning. Mary Ann told the staff that she just wanted to go to sleep. Just before eleven o'clock that night, Jackie went in to check on Mary Ann for the last time. The lights were down and the sheet was drawn over her head. Mary Ann was lying on her side, and Jackie was about to leave the room when she noticed that although her cardiac rhythm hadn't changed, the rate was faster than it was earlier.

Something told Jackie that Mary Ann was not simply sleeping. She pulled down the sheet with one hand and switched on the light with the other. Mary Ann was dripping with perspiration. Her eyes were rolled back in her head and she was blue. Jackie screamed for help when she saw the cable to the cardiac monitor. It was wrapped tightly twice around Mary Ann's neck.

Corinne ran into the room and found Jackie trying to pull the cable loose. She pulled the end off the monitor console, allowing it to be eased away from Mary Ann's neck. By this time Mary Ann began to come to. She started to cry, moaning that she couldn't even do this right. Physically, she was fine in a few minutes.

Jackie and Corinne were shaking. A few more minutes and there could have been a different ending. Mary Ann was transferred that night to the mental health unit, where she was put on a one to one suicide watch. Her vital signs were taken every fifteen minutes and she remained stable.

The ICU staff felt horrible, even though they knew they could not have done anything different. The psych unit was very tense, knowing what had almost happened to this young girl. And, in the middle was Mary Ann, a girl who felt that life had become so very unbearable that no life at all was better than the way she was now existing. Everyone lost that night.

IT SHOULDN'T HAVE BEEN

James Flannery had been ill for only a week. The pain had begun slowly, and over the next few days it had become progressively more severe. At first he thought it was just an upset stomach, maybe due to something he had eaten at that restaurant where he and his family had gone to celebrate the birth of his eighth grandchild.

Mr. Flannery had been a sick man. He had a long cardiac history, and had been in the hospital before for several vascular surgical procedures. His plumbing just wasn't so good, as he used to joke. But for the past three years he had felt better than ever. He enjoyed life and living.

Family discussions often included talks about living wills and the right to die. Mr. Flannery did not believe in keeping a person alive, if it appeared that it was dying that was being prolonged, rather than living. He had a living will, and was very familiar with advanced directives. That was perfectly clear. He didn't want his family to see him living on a ventilator, or as he put it, hanging on as a vegetable.

But this admission was different, somehow. All his previous problems had been cardiovascular. Now he just had this pain, this pain that just got worse and worse. It spread all over his abdomen, and he developed a fever. He was admitted to a medical floor and for whatever reason, just a few tests were done.

The next day, James Flannery became much worse. He seemed to have become septic. But his doctors didn't seem to want to become very aggressive. They discussed the situation with his family, since by this time James was almost unresponsive. Everyone knew James' feelings about being kept alive, and so he was made a DNR.

Something wasn't right. What was wrong with James Flannery? His nurses, on all shifts, felt uneasy. How could everyone just decide to let this man die? They didn't even have a diagnosis. Why was his abdomen so grossly distended? Why did he deteriorate so rapidly? What was going on?

By this time James Flannery was comatose. His temperature was very high and his respiratory rate was about fifty per minute. Now the doctors decided that maybe he had developed pulmonary emboli, and he should go to nuclear medicine for an emergency lung scan. This seemed crazy. Whether or not he had emboli, the nurses said, this was probably not the cause of his illness. If the disease was not being treated and he was being allowed to die, why put him through a lung scan? And to top it off, now they ordered a CT scan to follow. All of a sudden, three days after no attempt to diagnosis and treat, now he needed to have these procedures.

So, poor Mr. Flannery was brought down to nuclear medicine for a complete V/Q scan. The technologists knew he was a "no code" and probably dying. Connie stayed with him and held his hand during the test. By the time he came to CT, Mr. Flannery's respirations were about seventy per minute. The staff did not want to scan him. They put in a call to his doctor who said to do a simple and quick scan, but he "had to know what was going on."

Several minutes after the CT was started, Tony and Lois, the radiology nurses, watched his respirations become agonal. The technologists stopped the test. Lois went into the scanning room, and moved the table out. Lois and Tony each took one of Mr. Flannery's hands and began to speak quietly, telling him they were with him and he was not alone. Then James Flannery stopped breathing and died.

The CT staff called the medical unit. The floor nurse came down to radiology and started to cry as soon as she saw his body. Everyone knew why she cried, and it was not simply because a patient had died. Andrea cried from frustration and helplessness. The way this patient was managed was horrible. Could the doctors have done more? Definitely. Could the nurses have done more? Probably. Who lost? Everyone. Especially Mr. Flannery and his family.

Tony, Lois, and Andrea brought James Flannery back up to the floor. He was covered with a blanket and had an oxygen mask over his face, and he looked like he was sleeping. He seemed peaceful finally.

By the time the two nurses returned to the radiology department, the radiologist had read the lung scan. Normal. No pulmonary emboli. The half completed CT scan had also been read. Mr. Flannery had a small bowel obstruction causing all of his abdominal symptoms.

A small bowel obstruction. That was it. Maybe just adhesions. Maybe if he had been taken to surgery in time, the obstruction could have been released and the bowel would never had become gangrenous. Maybe he would have been ready for discharge by now.

There was no autopsy. There was no review. There was nothing but the final cause of death, listed simply as heart failure and cardiac arrest. A terrible end to this tragic case.

SMOKE

She could smell the smoke as soon as she got off the elevator. At first she thought there was a fire somewhere on the eighth floor, but something told her that this was different. Something worse.

It was three o'clock, the start of Pat's evening shift.

The corridor leading to the pulmonary ICU was deserted so she had nobody to ask what was happening. The odor got stronger as she got closer to the unit and she knew that whatever was going on was coming from inside those double doors.

As Pat entered the ICU, the first thing that hit her was the silence. The unit was full of residents, interns, and nurses, but nobody was doing anything. Nobody was talking. People were just standing around, looking at each other blankly.

It was a big unit and was very old. Instead of rooms or cubbies, the patients were all together in the one area separated only by dark green hospital curtains. All the curtains were pulled around the beds. Every single one. And the smell of smoke was hanging everywhere.

"What happened?" asked Pat out loud. "What happened?"

The day nurses didn't seem to hear her. Finally one of them shook her head. "A whole family was wiped out," she answered without any trace of emotion. Four of them were DOA and the mother and baby died up here. All from smoke inhalation."

Pat looked around and she noticed the crash cart in the middle of the unit, almost totally depleted. She walked over to the side of the unit which smelled the strongest and pulled back the curtain. There in the bed was a woman, obviously dead, with all her tubes and airways still in place. She walked over to the body and realized that she couldn't even tell the race of the woman, since her entire body was coated with black soot. Pat's eyes went to the suction bottle on the wall. The water in the bottle was jet black, showing that the same soot coating the body had been suctioned out of her lungs. No wonder she died.

Without thinking, Pat opened the next curtain. There right in the middle of the bed was a little baby, no more than nine months old and she was covered with the same horrible stuff. A tiny little endotracheal tube was sticking out of her mouth. The baby was also dead.

Pat slammed the curtain shut and took a big hard gulp of air. Then she opened it again and slowly walked over to the baby. The eyes were open but Pat could see that even the whites of her eyes looked brown. Soot. And the suction bottle water was black.

Turning around, Pat walked out to the nurses' station and realized she was shaking all over. By this time two of the day nurses began to talk. And once they started, they couldn't stop. The fire had apparently broken out just before dawn. By the time the fireman had gotten everyone out, it was daylight. The father and the other three kids were pronounced dead in the emergency department of the other hospitals, but the mother and baby had been brought here to the pulmonary ICU of this specialized pulmonary hospital. Nobody had been burned; they were all overcome by smoke. There were, of course, no smoke alarms.

The nurses hadn't even thought to get a crib for the baby and instead they had just thrown her into the big bed and had worked frantically for hours. The mother and baby had each arrested several times, until finally this last time their hearts were unable to be restarted.

Two other evening nurses had arrived by this time and Pat took them outside and told them what had happened. Ordinarily, the next shift would take over and do the post-mortem care, but today it was very obvious that the day nurses simply had to finish this. Somebody gave them a skimpy report on the other patients and the evening crew started to take care of the six remaining people. The patients who were awake knew what had happened and were scared to death. Two ladies were crying and one of the men had his face turned to the wall and his eyes shut tight. It was very sad.

The day shift did the post-mortem care together, crying as they washed some of the black stuff off the bodies. The Medical Examiner was waiting to take the bodies for autopsies and they knew they had to get them to the morgue as fast as possible. One of the day nurses suddenly announced that she was not going to separate the baby and her mother. She had an idea, and just let anyone try to stop her, she said. So they put a toe tag on each of the bodies and then they laid the dead baby in her mothers arms, tying them around her loosely with a soft piece of gauze. They then wrapped the two together in the same shroud pack and taped it closed. They put both tags outside of the shroud to let the morgue know that there were two bodies together inside.

Some how and some way this made those nurses feel better. That baby was not going down THERE alone. Mommy was with her. Nobody said a word. Nobody asked where the second body was. Everyone just knew and understood that this was the way it should be. And, somehow, that simple act of bringing the mother and her baby together for that final time made it seem just a little bit easier for everybody who worked so long and so hard to keep that family together.

ASPIRATION

Mr. Romero's abdomen had been a little distended when his family doctor admitted him, but by now it was three times as big. Mr. Romero had undergone a surgical procedure just six months earlier, and it looked like he had developed a partial bowel obstruction. It was most likely from adhesions, they said.

Nobody seemed too concerned, as this certainly was not an uncommon event after surgery. So, Mr. Romero was given nothing by mouth and started on intravenous fluids. A nasogatric tube was passed and was put to suction so as to keep the bowel empty and quiet. It was routine conservative medical treatment.

But, the belly continued to grow, and the tests showed the obstruction to be down lower in the intestine. It was not the small bowel after all, and the large intestine was becoming more and more distended. Mr. Romero obviously needed a cantor tube.

OK. No big deal. So he needed a cantor tube. Hopefully, that would decompress the intestine and surgery could be avoided. After all, nobody was too anxious to bring an old man back for a major abdominal procedure if there was another way.

Now, after three days in the hospital lots of old people start to get confused, and Mr. Romero was no exception. Kate finally got the cantor tube down him, and that was no easy job. The tube was in and put to suction, and now it was just time to wait and see if it would work. Mr. Romero kept forgetting where he was and what was going on, but he could easily be reoriented. Just to be on the safe side, Kate tied his hands loosely to the sides of the bed. It was just a reminder not to pull at the tube.

So the tube was in place but was not taped there, as is common practice with cantor tubes. After all, the whole purpose of that bag of mercury on the end of it was to weigh it down so it could move along in the bowel like a bolus of food during peristalsis. And, if it were anchored in place, it wouldn't go anywhere.

The last time Kate checked on Mr. Romero he was on his side as she had positioned him, fast asleep with the restraints in place. No problem. But when Kate came back a little later, she found Mr. Romero about to rip off the front of his face.

Somehow he had gotten his hands loose and decided it was time to pull out that big tube. He had managed to yank on the tube hard enough and long enough to work the big mercury filled bag up from the bowel into his stomach, and through his esophagus into his throat. Then he had either pulled it out or coughed and gagged the bag end out of his mouth. However, the other end was still coming out of his nose, right from the left nostril through which it had originally been inserted. So, Mr. Romero had a pulley system going. His left hand was pulling one end out of his mouth while the right one was pulling the other end out of his nose. He was jerking and tugging as hard as he could. The only way he could remove the tube that way was to detach the front of his face.

It was some sight and it took three people to pry his hands loose and calm Mr. Romero down. Kate knew she couldn't get that mercury bag back down his throat, so she decided that the only thing left to do was to cut the bag off from the twelve inches or so of the tube which was protruding from his mouth and then pull the tube up and out of his nose. So that's what she did.

Now it was back to square one. Mr. Romero was in bed with no tube and an abdomen which looked at least seven months pregnant. She had to insert another cantor tube and start again.

After giving him time to rest from his adventure, Kate came in with the tube. He seemed calm and cooperative and appeared to understand everything that Kate explained. Yeah, sure. He was fine when the tube was passed through his nose but when it was time to swallow the bag of mercury, Mr. Romero absolutely freaked out. He started yelling and gagging and fighting. Kate stopped what she was doing to try to calm him down, but Mr. Romero suddenly started to vomit. All this thick yellow stuff came up in his mouth. Kate grabbed an emesis basin and told Mr. Romero to spit it all up.

Mr. Romero did not listen, but instead got wilder and wilder. He began to scream at the top of his lungs at the same time that he was vomiting. Each time he took a big breath in to yell, he sucked in globs of the vomit along with the air. You could just hear that fluid being drawn down into his lungs. Kate began to yell for help as she grabbed for a suction tube to try to clear Mr. Romero's airway. But he kept fighting and screaming and vomiting, all at the same time.

Within a minute M. Romero finally got quiet, but by this time his eyes had rolled back in his head and he was blue. He was making little jerky movements with his chest but no air was moving. The staff called a code.

Kate couldn't function any more and she had to leave the room. The arrest team intubated Mr. Romero and suctioned what seemed like a quart of yellow vomitus out of his lungs. They tried for what seemed like forever and then the code was over. Mr. Romero was dead.

"I killed him. I killed him. I killed him," Kate kept repeating. "I really killed him. I can't believe I killed him." she said. There was nothing anyone could say to Kate. Mr. Romero had obviously died because he aspirated while the cantor tube was going down. That really was the reason and everybody including Kate knew it. It wasn't her fault, but that's exactly what happened.

That incident took place a long time ago. It would be great to say that Kate has passed many tubes since that time and that she has gotten over what happened that afternoon. But that's not the way it is. Kate has never inserted another cantor tube and says she never will. This one part of Kate's nursing skills which died that day with Mr. Romero. And Kate will always believe that she killed her patient.

PRACTICE

Over the past year, Joyce had really come to love this little man. He had been admitted to the oncology unit fairly often during his year of chemotherapy, and all of the staff had become part of his extended family.

Mr. Cohen had made it clear from the very start of his treatment just how he felt about his fight with cancer. He wanted to live as long as he was able to do so as a rational and thinking human being. He would never want to have his life extended by artificial means. He did not want to live on as a "vegetable," and if it ever came to that, his wish was to die peacefully and with dignity.

Mr. Cohen was seventy-five years old and had lived a very happy life. He had a large and loving family who visited often and who also had become close with the nurses. Knowing that the treatment he was getting was for the purpose of prolonging his life and not curing the disease, all of them together were comfortable in the care that Mr. Cohen was getting. All of them agreed that when the time came that things looked hopeless, he was to be kept comfortable and no heroics were to be done. Dying with dignity. That was the phrase used over and over again. Dying with dignity.

Joyce was working evenings during Mr. Cohen's last admission. This time things were very different. Rather than coming in for another three day course of chemotherapy, Mr. Cohen was admitted with respiratory difficulty. Tests showed a massive pleural effusion and ascites; fluid had formed around his lungs and all through his abdomen. It was obvious that the cancer had begun to spread rapidly and quite evident that Mr. Cohen was dying.

He wasn't the least bit afraid. Mr. Cohen, on the contrary, seemed almost relieved that now his future was more certain. He was going to see his beloved wife, he knew, who had died five years earlier. "It's really OK." Mr. Cohen told the nurses, with his usual gentle smile. "Don't worry about me. I'm at peace with this. Just let me be comfortable and let me keep my dignity."

Mr. Cohen was put on a morphine drip. He remained in a light sleep, but was comfortable when he was awakened. That was just the way he had told them so often that he wanted this to end. Everything was all right.

By the next day, Mr. Cohen had slipped into a coma. His attending physician had written a DNR order on his chart and had specified that nobody was to order any more tests or blood work. Mr. Cohen was to be allowed to drift off into his final sleep quietly, surrounded by his family. That's exactly what happened. Mr. Cohen died two days later, surrounded by his children and grandchildren and two of his favorite nurses. Joyce was there with him.

The family left after about ten minutes and Joyce returned to Mr. Cohen's private room to prepare his body for the morgue. When she came in with the shroud pack, she at first thought she had entered the wrong room. There were four medical residents standing around the bedside of Mr. Cohen. There were blood stains on the body and spattered over the sheets.

"What are you doing?" whispered Joyce, not comprehending just what it was that she was seeing.

"We're practicing central IV lines and doing pericardial taps," answered one of the residents without even looking up. As he spoke those words, Joyce watched him push the big long cardiac needle right into Mr. Cohen's chest, aiming for the sac around the heart. For just a few moments, Joyce was frozen She couldn't move and she couldn't speak.

Then suddenly, she ran towards the bed, screaming out loud, "Stop that! Get away from him!"

One of the doctors looked up at her as if there were something wrong with her. "What do you mean?" he asked, genuinely surprised. "How are we supposed to learn these things if we don't practice? This is a teaching hospital. So what's the problem?"

Before she could respond, he took his big long introducer needle, and pushed it deep into the right side of the chest, looking for the vena cava.

Joyce lunged forward, grabbing the doctor's hand and pulling the needle out of the chest. "Get away! Get away!" she screamed at him. The resident, his face suddenly red, began to physically fight with Joyce over the needle, which was dripping with blood. If anyone had walked into the room at that moment, they realized later, what they would have witnessed would have been unbelievable.

The rest of the people in the room started to scream at the doctor and the nurse to stop it before one of them stabbed the other with that big contaminated needle. The resident, cursing loudly, somehow got the needle away from Joyce and threw it down on the floor. Then he stormed out of the room. The three other residents, calling Joyce a lunatic and a crackpot, followed him. Joyce backed up and sat down in the chair in the corner of the room. Then she began to cry. Had this sort of stuff been going on all the time in her hospital without her even knowing it? Is that the way things are done in teaching hospitals? Are all the patients allowed to be guinea pigs?

Joyce got a basin of warm water and began to wash Mr. Cohen's body. Dark blood was trickling from all the holes in his chest. Joyce, with tears running down her face, put pressure on all the wound sites without really knowing why. She knew there were no clotting mechanisms working any more in this dead body but she pressed anyway, and eventually the blood just stopped.

"I'm so sorry. I'm so sorry, Mr. Cohen," Joyce kept repeating. "I let you down. I didn't mean to, Mr. Cohen."

She changed the bloody linen and took it out of the room, as if removing it could take back what had happened in there.

At the end of the shift, Joyce went home. She was still in a state of shock, but she knew she had a lot of work ahead of her. She didn't know how and she didn't know when, but she knew one thing. Joyce was going to see that this type of thing was not going to be routine practice. At least not in her hospital. She owed that to Mr. Cohen and all the other Mr. Cohens to come. And, she would succeed or she wouldn't be a hospital nurse anymore. Of that much, she definitely was certain.

THE REASON

It wasn't really a lump she felt. It was more of a thickening. She knew she had cystic breasts and she did routine self exams each month. There was no history of breast cancer in her family and, after all, she was only thirty-five years old. So she really wasn't worried.

And, it hurt. It just felt sore. She had read somewhere that breast cancer isn't painful, so that was something else to put her at ease. Her mammogram six months earlier was okay, except for the cysts which she knew she had. That's the reason she had gone for the first mammo anyway. Everything was fine, they said.

But Ruth was a little uneasy. She knew what those cysts felt like, and this just felt different to her. So being the careful person that she always was, Ruth made an appointment with her doctor, the same gynecologist whom she had been seeing for years.

"I don't feel anything," he told her. "The mammogram was normal and there's nothing there. Besides breast cancer doesn't hurt," he told her. "You women are so jittery. You read too much. Relax. You're fine. It's just hormones that make you feel sore."

Since the doctor had told Ruth exactly what she was hoping to hear, she was happy and relieved. After all, she told herself, he was the doctor. He knew more than she did. Maybe she didn't like the way he spoke to her, but that wasn't what mattered. The point was that she was okay, and the doctor said that she was.

Over the next few months, the soreness never went away. That was a little strange, Ruth thought. Usually any feelings like that got better or worse depending on the time of the month. But this time it stayed the same. The breast still felt different to her. There still was no lump, but the whole top part felt funny. Thicker and harder.

Even though Ruth knew the doctor was probably going to brush her off again, she called him. She spoke to his nurse this time, who Ruth had always liked, and she explained everything to her. Later that afternoon, the nurse called her back and said the doctor had scheduled her for another mammogram. This would put her mind at ease, the doctor had said.

But the results were far from reassuring. The radiologist had called the area which Ruth pointed out "suspicious," and now Ruth was scheduled to see a surgeon. The appointment was made for the following afternoon. Ruth didn't get much sleep that night. When the surgeon told her that he thought the area should be biopsied, Ruth was ready for that. She had known this was coming. When the biopsy result showed a malignancy, Ruth expected that too. She just knew.

154

After a second opinion and reviewing Ruth's options with her and her husband, Ruth underwent a simple mastectomy and dissection of the nodes under her arm. The news from that procedure was not good. The pathologist found five lymph nodes had already been infiltrated with cancer cells. A bone scan showed two spots in her spine where the cancer had spread.

From that day on, Ruth began her war against cancer. She was treated at a big cancer center. Chemotherapy and radiation combined with holistic medicine began. Ruth underwent two autologous bone marrow transplants. Her fight lasted almost four years, but the cancer came back. Again and again, when she thought she just might have licked the disease, it showed up again in another place.

Ruth lost her battle with breast cancer, but she fought hard and long. All the time, she knew that if her gynecologist had listened to her back then, her odds may have been better. During her struggle, she said over and over again that women must not let themselves be intimidated by doctors who call them hysterical or tell them they overreact. Breast cancer does not always behave like the books say it does. It can strike younger women and it can hurt. When Ruth knew she was dying, she said she wanted that to be her legacy. She wanted women to know that they, and not their doctors, know their own bodies.

By speaking out this way, Ruth said, they may just save their own lives. Surely Ruth, in her message to others, must have helped many people. If there has to be a reason, maybe, just maybe, that was why Ruth had to die.

EPILOGUE

Nobody, except for other nurses, really knows what it means to be a nurse. We nurses are special. We share the heartache and the joy, the tears and the smiles. We are the hands to hold and the shoulders to cry on. We give and receive those first hugs of relief and are present for the long-awaited good news, or the dreaded bad news.

We are privileged to be part of another person's pain or joy. There is no other profession that allows such closeness with our fellow man. We give a lot of ourselves, but we get so much back. Nursing is a natural high.

Every nurse knows the feeling of having a "good day." We know it when we have helped an incontinent gentleman regain his dignity, or when we have made a post-operative patient comfortable, both physically and emotionally. We know it when we have spent time in the Emergency Department with the family of a critically injured child, assuring them that everything possible is being done. There is no feeling, for a nurse, like the satisfaction of helping. Of course we don't always have good days, but those good ones more than make up for those that are not so good.

Nurses share something so unique, so special, that it is very difficult to explain it to an outsider. We laugh at the same things. With just a look, we can communicate a feeling about a patient or a doctor. We have a special type of intuition and of understanding of what should be and what could happen. It doesn't matter if the nurse works in the operating room, in a clinic, or in the home --- there's just something very distinct about all nurses. We understand each other.

Nurses remain nurses forever. It's in our blood. We are the best part of the helping professions; we are the most special, the elite.

We are nurses and we should be very proud.

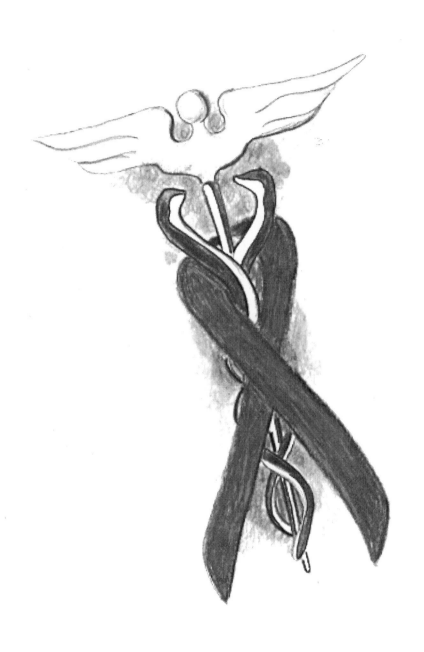